# PREGNANCY DIET
## A Practical Guide for Busy Women

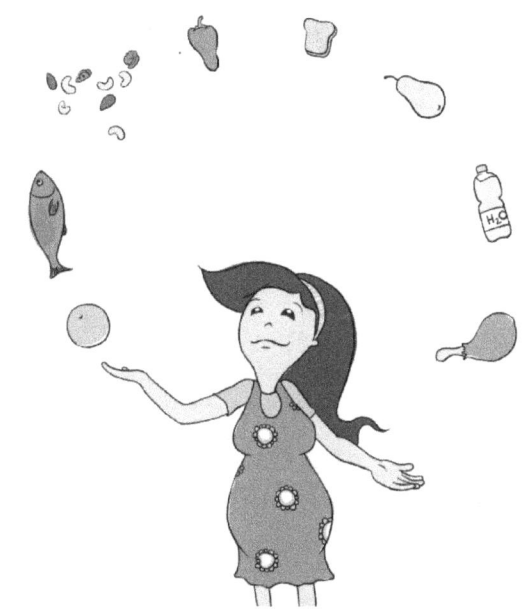

## Written By: Einat L. K.

Edited By: Robert Shveytser
Pregnant woman illustrations By: Leda Vaneva

ISBN No. 978-1630220686

First Printing, 2014

Printed in the United States of America

www.MyPregnancyToolkit.com

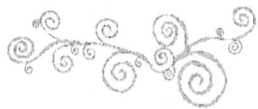

By purchasing this book you've taken the **first step** in eating nutritious food that will help you keep a healthy pregnancy for you and your child. The **next step** would be to read it and use the techniques it introduces. I believe that the results will make you happy.

This book was written with love and care, to support you in managing a healthy pregnancy diet in your busy life.

If you like this book, please stop by and review it at:

Your success means a lot to me.

If you have a comment or question, please contact me at my email address:

contact@myPregnancyToolkit.com

My wish is for you to have a healthy pregnancy accompanied by good nutrition.

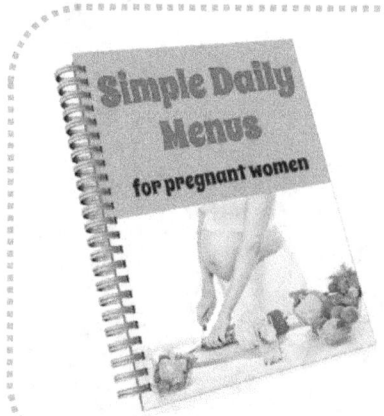

Scan the following code to grab a complimentary copy of your special gift for busy women. *"Simple Daily Menus"* – suggestions for different meals throughout the day.

# TABLE OF CONTENTS

# PUBLISHER'S NOTES

# DEDICATION

This book is dedicated to my mother, who taught me to always search for simple and easy solutions to solve the various challenges I encounter in life.

# CHAPTER 1 - INTRODUCTION

**Greetings!**

I want to congratulate you on deciding to take care of your own and your baby's health during your pregnancy. By picking up this book you have taken an important first step towards a healthy and happy nine months. You are now ready to begin preparing food that will help your child develop during the coming months.

Cooking can be a tedious chore, one that many busy working women don't have much time for. Add to that the complication of having to think about what to eat and what not to eat while pregnant. There are many different recommendations to follow and many warnings to consider about what is good for the development of the fetus.

This book will help you by providing a simple and easy method for preparing healthy and nutritious food that will benefit both you and your growing baby. It will also give you tips to help you get through the pregnancy, as well as show shortcuts to a healthy diet.

Your baby depends on you to provide all the nutrients he needs to develop properly. The quality of the food you consume during your pregnancy determines your baby's health now and during his whole life. Nutritious food can make the difference between illness and health.

By consuming food that is good for you, you can ease any potential negative symptoms of pregnancy and have a healthy childbirth without complications. Food can have a great impact on your mood and can even affect your ability to breast feed your baby. Caring for your health and thinking about your nutrition intake is therefore very important.

After reading this book, you will have a method for making healthy food in a quick and simple way. You will know what foods to eat during your pregnancy and how your meals can help you through this mentally- and physically-straining time.

Imagine yourself eating nutritious foods that helps your child develop naturally and gives you a healthy body. **Your pregnancy will be easy, your test results excellent and you will be filled with energy.**

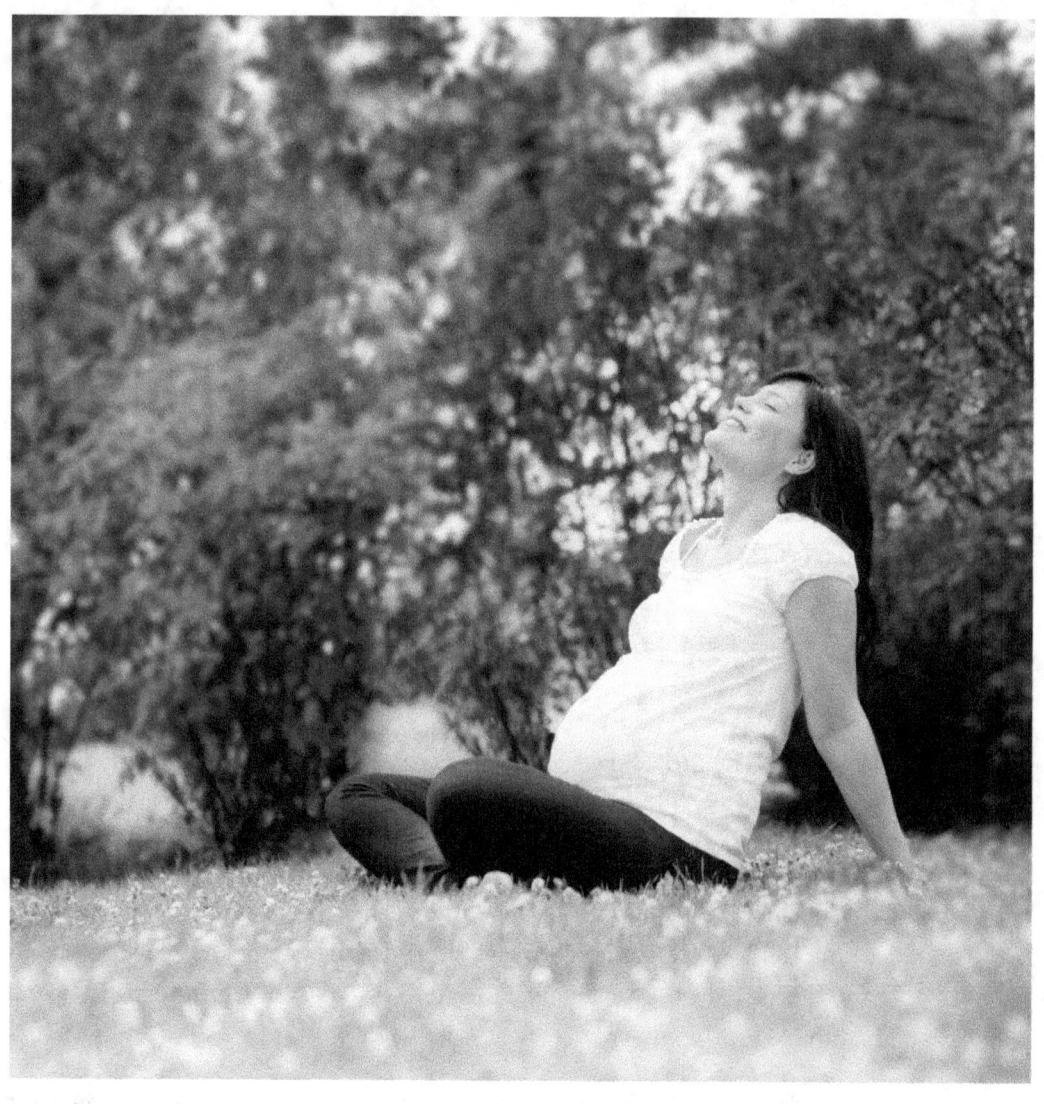

The meals at which we will look during this book will provide you with all the essential ingredients to help both your self and your child feel good. Your mood will be better and you will be filled with energy. You'll no longer have to worry about what you can or cannot eat and instead will know what is good for you and your baby.

There are many concerns about nutrition during pregnancy. You may be too busy to think about what to eat or maybe you don't like to cook at all. Perhaps you don't know which foods have better nutritional value and which ingredients you should be eating to help your baby develop properly so he can have a healthy start in life. You may be fearful that foods you are now consuming could even be dangerous or harmful to your child.

Due to the risks involved, this is not a worry that should be ignored. An unhealthy diet during the early development can cause illnesses and defects throughout your child´s life. **It is important that you take your concerns seriously and think carefully about what to eat.**

This book will help you find out which nutrients your baby needs for a healthy future development. You will not only learn what foods to avoid, but also find a quick and easy method of preparing food that is beneficial to you and your child. Just as important, you will be cooking meals that taste good. After reading this book, you will be able to go into the kitchen with confidence and knowledge on how to make simple, healthy meals that will benefit you and your child.

I was in your situation when I was pregnant with my oldest daughter. All the different recommendations and warnings filled me with uncertainty and doubt, and I constantly worried that I was eating something that could potentially harm my baby´s development.

I was filled with questions but had few answers. How would I get through the pregnancy? Would I feel good? What *could* I eat and what could harm my growing child?

I knew from the start that nutrition was important, and I knew I should be eating healthy and nutritious food. After wondering and worrying for a long time, I began to research the subject in depth. I was able to make a list of foods I should eat while pregnant and this eventually became a menu for pregnant women. As one who hates cooking, I was looking for easy solutions and simple meals.

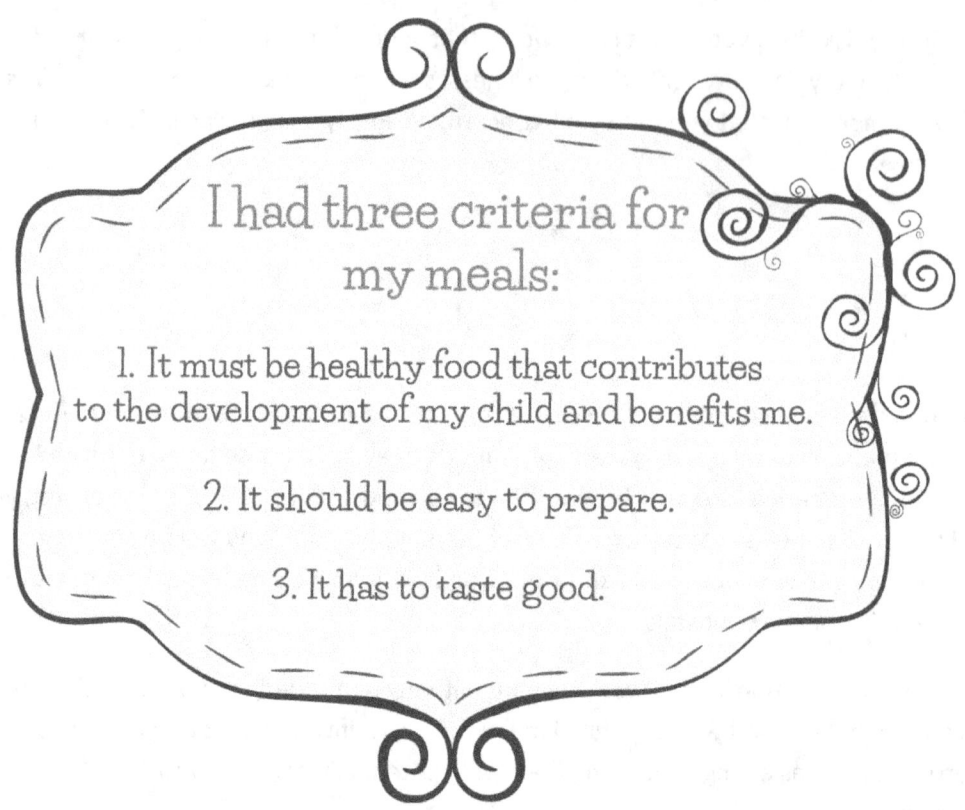

I had three criteria for my meals:

1. It must be healthy food that contributes to the development of my child and benefits me.

2. It should be easy to prepare.

3. It has to taste good.

These criteria allowed me to create a list of simple and delicious meals that consist of foods recommended for pregnant women. My pregnancy went very well and my daughter was delivered healthy and on time by natural birth. As a bonus, I never did spend too much time in the kitchen.

The idea for this book arose from my desire to pass on my knowledge to other women who might be struggling to figure out what to eat during their pregnancies. I want to share my method of preparing fast and easy meals at home which would help you and your child.

I believe that all women should be concerned about proper nutrition, not just during their pregnancies, but in their everyday lives (though that is the subject for another book). Food has the power to affect your mood and your body. It provides your growing baby with proper nutrition and helps him develop into a strong and healthy child.

So take the power into your own hands and read this book. Start eating healthy today, for the sake of both your child and you.

# Chapter 2- How can healthy nutrition affect your pregnancy and your baby's development?

## The Effects of Poor Nutrition

Your child is completely dependent on the nutrients in the food you consume during pregnancy. What you eat will directly contribute to your child's development and determine his current and future health. It is therefore vital that you eat food which is healthy for both of you.

**Improper nutrition can cause problems during pregnancy and lead to deficiencies later in life.** Some food might contain bacteria that can seriously harm your baby's development and even prove **fatal**.

Poor nutrition in the mother can cause **placental abruption**. The placenta is attached to the uterine wall and provides your growing child with food and oxygen. Placental abruption is the separation of placenta from this wall before birth. If this happens, your child might not receive the oxygen or nutrition he needs.

The most common cause for placental abruption is trauma to the abdominal area, but a lack of nutrition or water can also pose a serious risk. If your blood volume fails to keep up with the growing placenta, your blood flow behind the placenta slows down and may cause an abruption. Drink plenty of water and consume enough calories to make sure you are not at risk.

Poor nutrition can also make the **placenta fragile**, which can cause postpartum hemorrhage and require blood transfusions.

Iron helps create hemoglobin, which carries oxygen to your cells, and a deficiency of iron causes anemia with symptoms such as tiredness, dizziness and weakness. While pregnant, you are more at risk of iron deficiency since your blood amount increases by almost 50 percent and needs more iron to produce hemoglobin. Make sure to consume iron-rich food such as red meat, egg yolk, beans and spinach and take a supplement with at least 18 to 27 milligrams of iron per day.

Poor nutrition can **cause the perineum to lose some of its flexibility**. This can cause significant tears by the delivery of even an average or small-size baby.

Proper nutrition can **ensure that labor does not begin too early** and a healthy body will help you through the physical trial of childbirth. It will give you energy postpartum and ensure you have the energy to deal with a newborn.

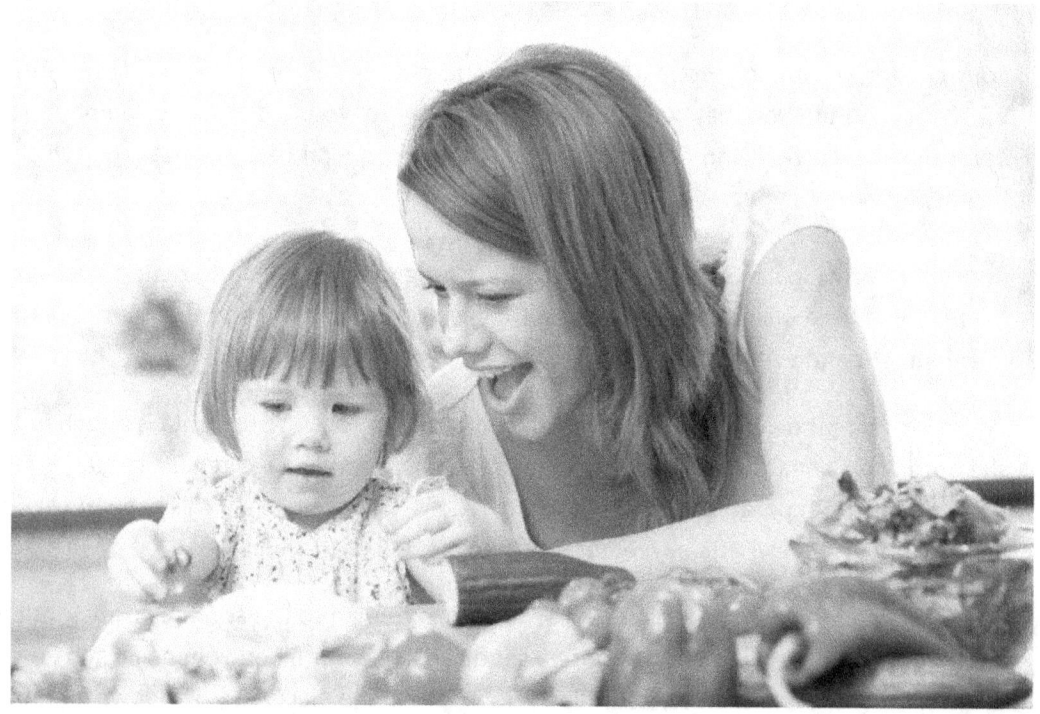

Healthy foods that include whole grains, vegetables, fruit and protein strengthen your immune system and make it easier for both you and your growing child to defeat infections. It can aid in the production of breast milk, ensuring you have plenty of healthy milk ready for when your child is born.

You can also relieve any swelling of feet and ankles with a diet rich on potassium which includes vegetables and a lot of liquids. Once your pregnancy is over, having stuck to a **healthy diet will pay off by giving you less weight to lose**.

The most important reason for expectant mothers to eat healthy, however, is the fact that **poor nutrition can damage your child's health**. Folates found in lemons, bananas and leafy vegetables, among other foods, contribute to the healthy development of your child´s spine as well as his brain. Healthy nutrition can also keep your child from developing Type 2 Diabetes and obesity.

A healthy diet during your first trimester is crucial for a proper development of your baby´s organs. Studies have shown that consuming a lot of proteins, fluids, whole grains and fresh fruit reduces the risk of cardiovascular illnesses in your child.

Some of the things we eat and drink could be directly harmful to your child, of which alcohol and caffeine are the most obvious. Fish high in mercury should be avoided, as well as soft cheeses that may contain Listeria.

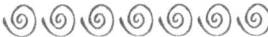

*Anne didn´t read about nutrition during her pregnancy, but stuck to her tough workout-plan without adding any food to her diet. She didn't know she was supposed to put on a little weight during pregnancy and had no idea the food she was eating would affect the development of her child. Her delivery went fine, but a while later her son had several seizures which were attributed to poor nutrition during early development. Fortunately her son recovered and is now healthy, but Anne has learned the hard way the importance of healthy and proper nutrition.*

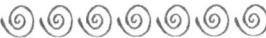

## Two Simple Principles For Proper Nutrition

**There are two simple principles to adhere to if you want to give your child the best possible start in life:**

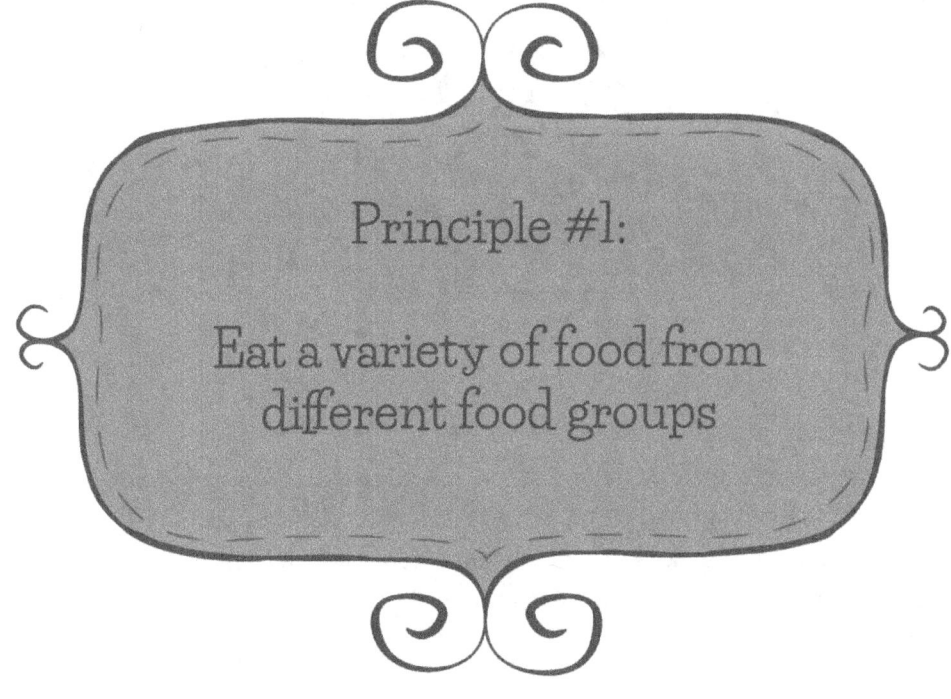

Principle #1:

Eat a variety of food from different food groups

- **Fruits and vegetables:** contain beta carotene which is beneficial to your baby´s cell development, eye-sight and immune system; vitamin C, which is essential to a good development of teeth and bones; potassium, which helps control blood pressure; folic acid, which prevents neural tube defects and can help promote a healthy birth weight.
- **Whole grains:** Bread and cereal contain folic acid, iron and fiber.
- **Meat, beans, fish, eggs and nuts:** Protein from red or white meat or beans is necessary for creating new tissue and will promote the healthy development of your child; fish contains plenty of omega-3 fatty acids which are critical for the neurodevelopment and may help with a healthy birth weight; eggs are similarly rich in fatty acids and other important nutrients.
- **Dairy products:** Cheese, milk, yogurt and cream contain calcium, protein, vitamin D and phosphorous which are important for the development of your baby´s teeth, bones, muscles, heart and nerves.

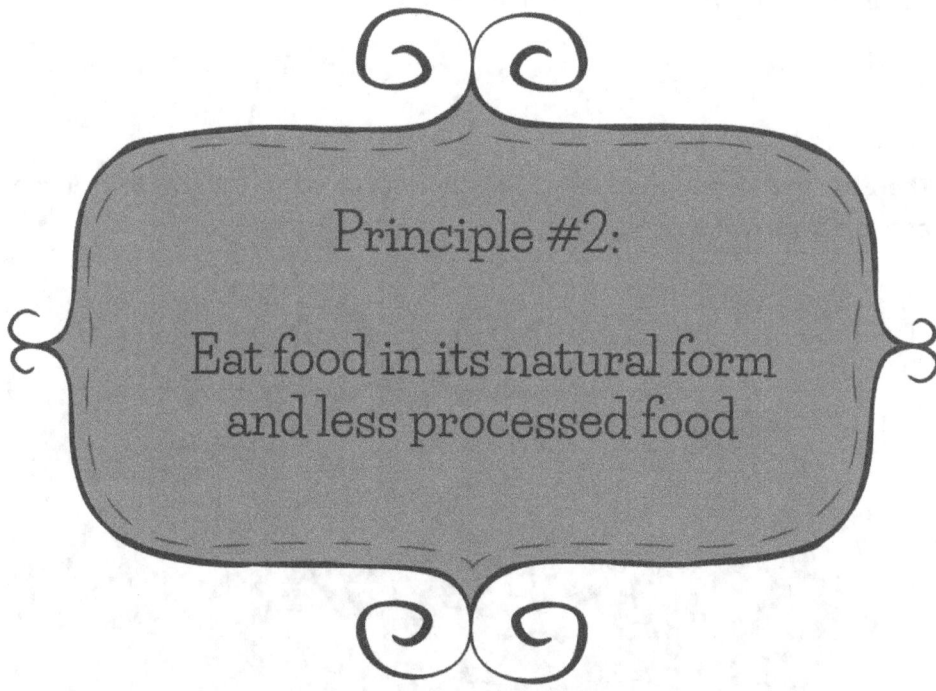

Principle #2:

Eat food in its natural form and less processed food

- Eating less processed food helps you to avoid trans fats, refined carbohydrates and additives such as sugar, sodium, preservatives and colorings. Cutting these from your diet can help you lose weight and gain more energy. Unprocessed food contains more vitamins and nutrients that will help both you and your baby during pregnancy.

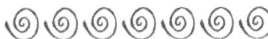

*Louise knew about the importance of nutrition but thought it didn´t apply to her. Her family had a history of healthy children, and she thought she as well was sure to deliver a healthy child without complications. Her diet consisted mainly of fast food and soda, and she began to eat more of it since she now felt she could "eat for two". Her son was born full-term but she was later warned that he was at a risk of developing diabetes and obesity.*

*The issue prompted Louise to research diets further and for her second pregnancy she ate only healthy food which would provide her with the right nutrition. Her youngest son was born healthy and had no issues with weight.*

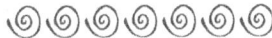

*"Better to eat a dry crust of bread with peace of mind than have a banquet in a house full of trouble."*

*~ Proverbs*

# Chapter 3- How can your mind affect your eating habits?

## The Power Of The Mind

Many women think they need to prepare themselves in order to begin eating healthy food. They might feel they need to plan a diet, learn how to cook or clear a lot of time in their busy schedules for just one meal. At this point, eating healthy becomes a chore, a complex and complicated matter better abandoned before it's even begun.

When you are pregnant, you no longer have the choice of putting the matter aside. Now you are responsible not only for your own body, but for the current and future well-being of your child. What you put in your mouth does not concern just you anymore.

**Don´t worry, the complex issue of diets is about to get a lot more simple.**
Instead of starting with what goes into your mouth, let´s look at what goes into your mind.

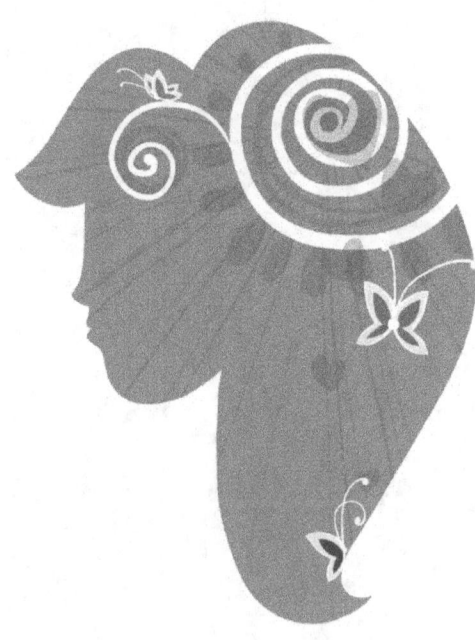

Your mind is a powerful ally in your pursuit for a healthy diet. Strengthening your mind and working towards eating well is a winning combination.

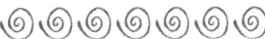

*Loreen was brought up on vegetables as a member of a vegan family. She was always healthy, but to her there was something missing in her diet. As soon as she moved out, she discovered all of the things she had been missing out on before. Now she switched from healthy fruits and vegetables to fast foods, fatty meat and ice cream.*

*Her weight increased steadily, but she could never imagine going back to eating only vegetables, like she had when she was a child. She resented traditional healthy food and would often describe herself as proud of her weight.*

*Only when she learned that she was pregnant did she stop to think about what she was eating and how it was affecting her body. Her doctors warned her of the risk of blood clots, and she realized she needed to make a change if she wanted to stay safe and live to see her child.*

*She decided to make a change in her view regarding vegetables. Instead of being her enemy, they became her ally and an important part of her diet. Gradually she became healthier and gave birth to a healthy baby girl. The switch in her mind persisted. She continued to eat well and felt her energy levels rise even when she was a new mother.*

*Her mind helped her make the change from unhealthy to healthy food. Strengthening your mind helps you make a commitment and stick to it, which is important when your will to eat healthy falters.*

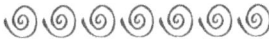

## TOOLS FOR HELPING YOU STRENGTHEN YOUR MIND
**There are several valuable tools to help you strengthen your mind:**

### POSITIVE AFFIRMATIONS
Thinking positively about healthy food and healthy living can help you get through the worst periods of doubt and weakness. Use the following affirmations to strengthen your resolve and feel good about the new, healthier you. Repeat these sentences often to yourself and feel the difference:

- I am fit, healthy and attractive
- My baby will be healthy because I eat healthy
- I only eat healthy food

17

- I know how to take care of myself during my pregnancy
- I eat with discipline
- I give my baby proper nutrition

You can learn more about how to use the positive affirmation technique in my book *How to Reduce Pregnancy Stress Using the Positive Affirmations Technique*

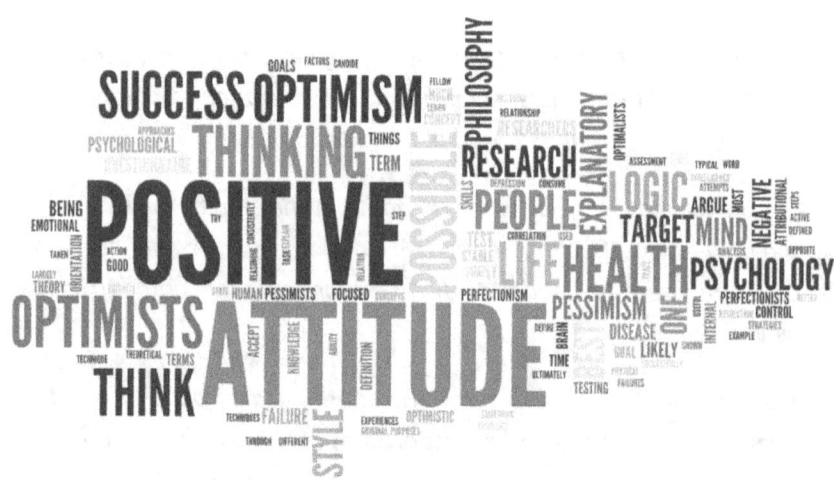

## VISION BOARD

A vision board is a poster board where you paste (create a collage) images from various magazines or the internet for inspiration. The idea is that when you surround yourself with positive images, your mind will be set on making changes for the better.

All you need is a poster board, a stack of magazines and glue. Cut out images that inspire you to eat healthy. Perhaps they are of you as you would like to look in the future, with a healthy body. Perhaps they are of the healthy meals you will learn to cook. Some might represent your future baby, who is happy and healthy.

## VISION MOVIE

A vision movie is a practical tool to fulfill different purposes in your life. It is a personal movie done with you, by you and for you. Define your wishes and goals to yourself. Make a video where you tell yourself why you want to eat healthy and how you will feel when you accomplish this. It should combine positive statements to yourself, pictures of your dreams and inspirational music of your choice.

The movie transmits to your consciousness the image of how you want life to be and internalizes it in your mind. This will allow you to visualize your new and healthier lifestyle and will make the change a part of your everyday life.

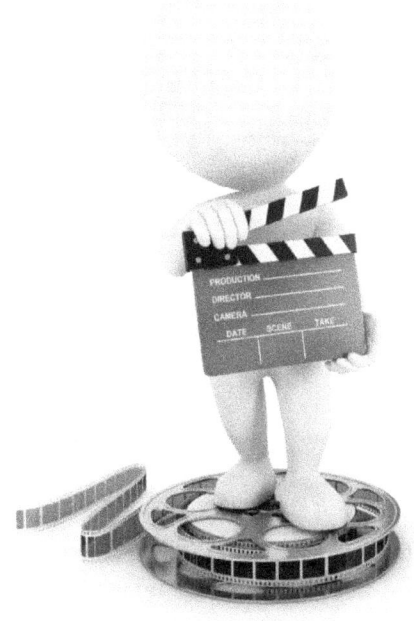

## SEINFELD´S METHOD OF PERSISTENCE

This is a simple method to encourage you to act every day to improve your life. Actor and comedian Jerry Seinfeld devised this method for himself in order to be more productive in his writing. He created a unique calendar system which you can use for any area in your life in order to achieve your goals.

Begin with setting your goal: to eat healthy. Take a month-long or a year-long calendar and put it up on a prominent wall. For every day that you follow your new goal and eat healthy with your baby in mind, put a big, red X over that day. Now all you have to do is not break the chain of red Xs.

The idea behind the method is that if you skip one day, it´s much easier to skip the next. By trying to earn the X and not break the chain, you also develop a habit of eating healthy food which is good not only during your pregnancy, but for the rest of your life.

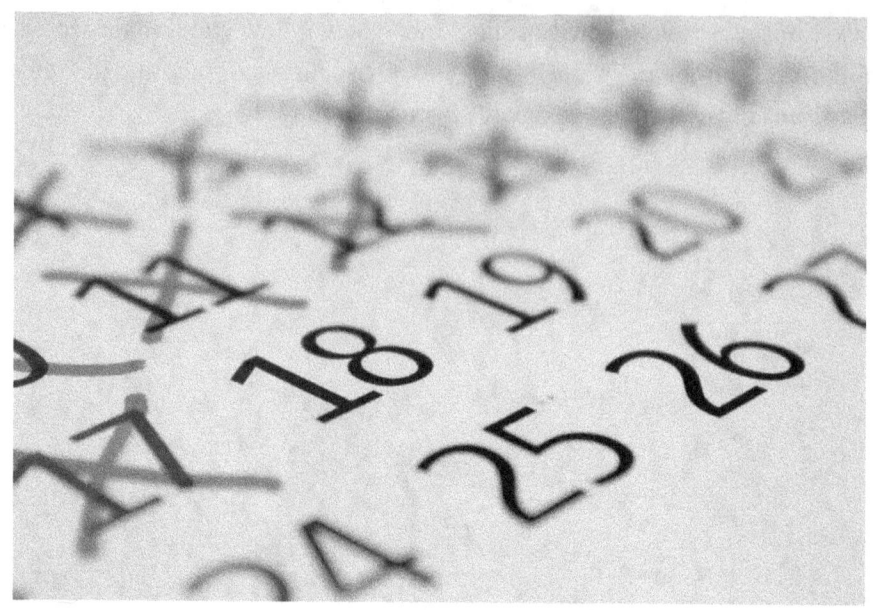

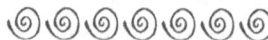

Amanda had never been able to stick to a diet, so when she was pregnant with her first child she thought she had to struggle with a guilty conscience for nine months. At first, she found it very difficult to stick to a routine of healthy meals. She was used to fast food and TV dinners  and had little spare time to spend in the kitchen.

She learned about the vision board from a friend and set one up in her hallway. As she left her house to do her food shopping, the last thing she would see were pictures of healthy meals and a smiling baby. These images continually inspired her to make a change, and instead of microwave dinners she would return from the store with bags full of vegetables, fruits and whole-grain bread. Amanda had a healthy pregnancy and looked fitter than ever just a few months after her daughter was born.

**Changing your mindset is an important step, but it must be combined with concrete actions. This is something we will look at in the next chapter in the book.**

*"We are shaped by our thoughts; we become what we think. When the mind is pure, joy follows like a shadow that never leaves."*

*~ Buddha*

# CHAPTER 4- WHICH NUTRIENTS ARE RECOMMENDED FOR PREGNANT WOMEN AND IN WHICH FOODS CAN YOU FIND THEM?

The first step to planning a healthy menu is finding out which nutrients you and your baby require. Your body is changing, and proper nutrition will help it deal with the increased demands of pregnancy. At the same time, your baby will need a specific set of nutrients to develop properly.

Sometimes it can be difficult to get all the nutrients through a healthy diet alone. Because of this, you should probably take vitamin and mineral pregnancy supplements that will ensure you meet your recommended daily intake. It is advisable to consult with your doctor before deciding on any supplements, however, as some vitamins can be dangerous during this time.

Folic acid, also called folate, is vitamin B. It helps prevent birth defects in the baby´s brain and spinal cord and plays an important role in the production of red blood cells. Since these types of birth defect occur during the first few weeks of pregnancy, it is important that the mother has enough folates before conception and the first few months afterwards. Supplements which contain folic acid have also been shown to reduce the risk of heart defects, cleft lips and urinary tract anomalies.

Here is a detailed list of the foods you need during your pregnancy. You should choose from the items and form a balanced diet that also fits your taste preference.

Remember to adhere to the two principles mentioned in the first chapter:

Principle #1: Eat a variety of foods from different food groups.

Principle #2: Eat food in its natural and not processed form.

*FRUITS AND VEGETABLES*

Fruits and vegetables are full of nutrients and fibers, and should be an important part of your diet while you are pregnant.

**Why is it important?** Vitamins in fruits and vegetables are needed for the cell and tissue development of your child; they boost the immune system and are crucial to your baby's bones and teeth.

**Examples of food**: Grapefruits, oranges, lemons, pears, pineapple, asparagus, avocados, beets, peppers.

**Consumption suggestions**: Fruits, both fresh and dried, are excellent snacks. Vegetables can be eaten as a part of a cooked meal or as healthy salads.

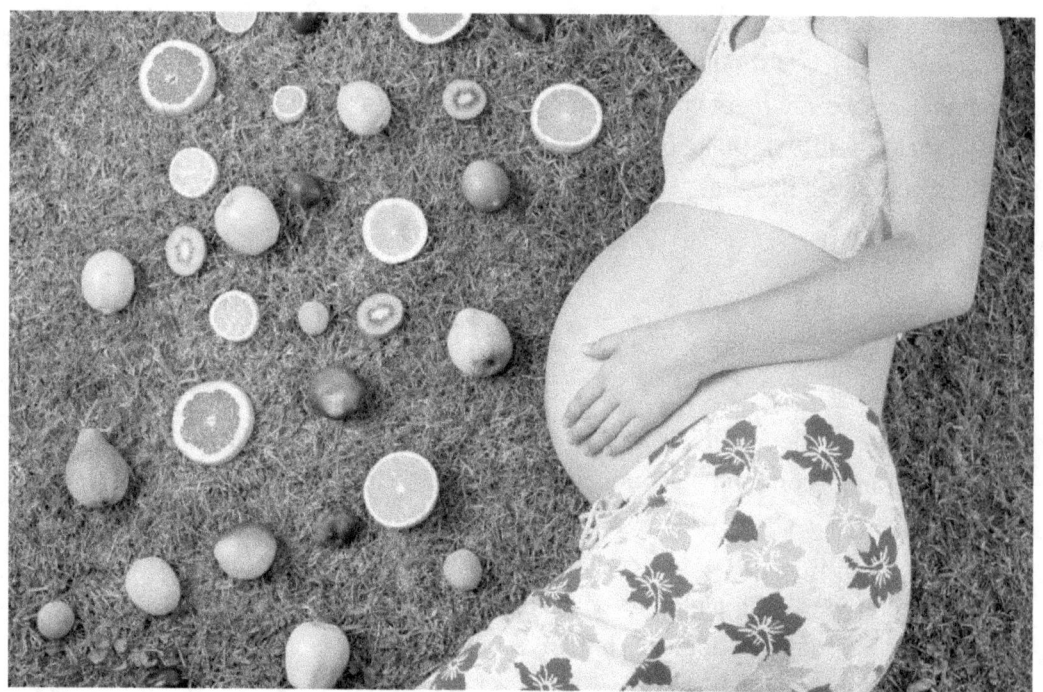

*WHOLE GRAINS*

Whole grains and food made from whole grains contain all the essential and natural ingredients of the entire grain seed.

**Why is it important?** Grains contain many valuable nutrients such as iron, selenium, magnesium and vitamins B1, B2, folic acid and niacin. These foods boost the development of your baby and the placenta.

**Examples of food**: Rice, oatmeal, bread, pancakes, noodles, pasta.

**Consumption suggestions**: Popcorn is a healthy snack which contains whole grain, as is quinoa. Eat a healthy, whole-grain breakfast or a whole-grain pasta salad for lunch.

### PROTEIN-RICH FOODS
Proteins perform many important functions in the body, such as replicating DNA and driving metabolic reactions.

**Why is it important?** Protein and their amino acids help build human cells. Your baby will need a lot of proteins to develop properly, so make sure to have a protein-rich diet during your pregnancy.

**Examples of food**: Eggs, red meat, cheese, lentils, tofu, yogurt, chicken.

**Consumption suggestions**: Choose protein-rich meals or add some grated cheese to your salad.

### FOOD RICH IN MONOUNSATURATED FATS
There are good fats and bad fats, and while pregnant you should try to eat the fats that are healthy for you. Monounsaturated fats are found in safflower, olives, canola and peanuts, for example.

**Why is it important?** Monounsaturated fats are considered the healthiest fats for you and are good for lowering your cholesterol. They often contain vitamin E, which is an important antioxidant.

**Examples of food**: Peanuts, olives or olive oil, avocados, hazelnuts, pistachios.

**Consumption suggestions**: Eat nuts as a healthy snack and include avocado in your salads. Use olive- or safflower oil instead of other products.

### FOODS RICH IN OMEGA-3 AND OMEGA-6 FATTY ACIDS
Fatty acids are the building blocks of fats, which are vital nutrients.

**Why is it important?** Omega-3 can help prevent blood clotting, build cell membranes and support general cell health. Omega-6 improve brain function, promote a healthy skin and help muscle growth and muscle repairs.

**Examples of food**: Omega-3: fatty fish such as salmon, anchovies or trout, flaxseed oil or walnut oil. Omega-6: vegetable oils such as sunflower or soybean oil, avocados, nuts, seeds, animal meat, egg yolks and shellfish.

**Consumption suggestions**: Switch to organic meat and milk or meat from cows feeding in pastures, since the grass they eat boost omega-3. Eat walnuts and include salmon in your lunch salad.

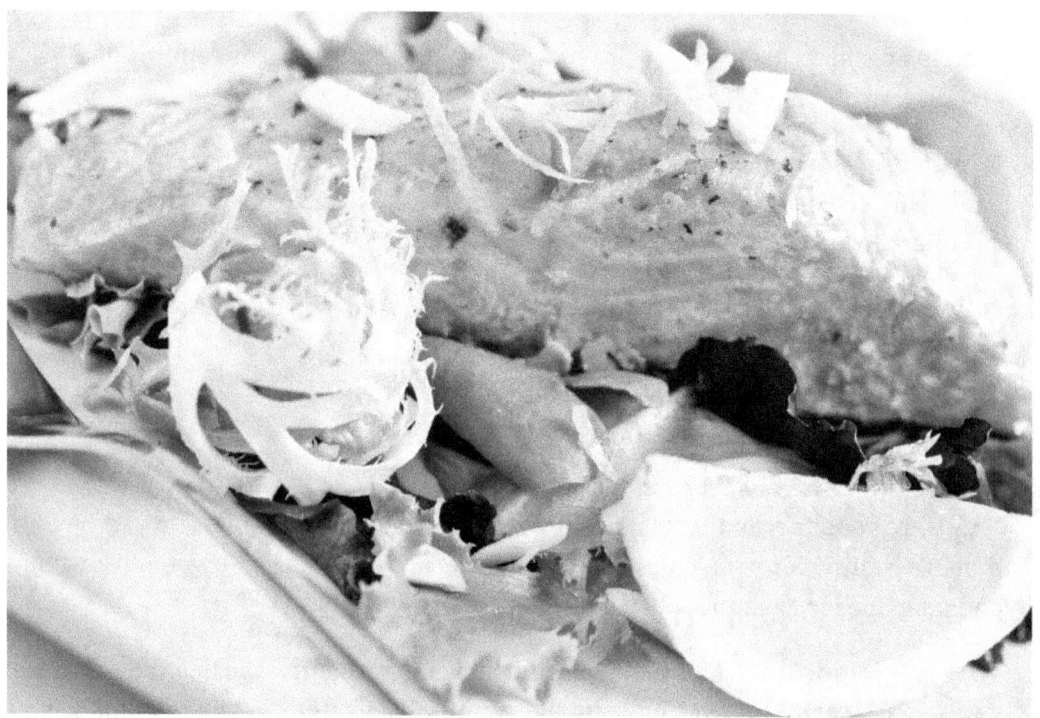

## CALCIUM

Calcium is an important part of any diet, and even more so while you are pregnant.

**Why is it important?** Calcium helps the development of your baby's bones and teeth, heart, nerves and muscles. It is important that you consume enough calcium while pregnant, as your baby will otherwise draw it from your bones which could cause you difficulties later on.

**Examples of food**: Yogurt, cheese, sardines, orange juice, tofu, salmon, spinach, turnips, sesame seeds.

**Consumption suggestions**: Make sure to include dairy products in your menu, use tahini as a salad dressing and eat meals fortified with calcium. Tap water can contain 135 mg of calcium per liter. Don't consume more than 2,500 mg of calcium as this can increase your risk of kidney stones and may cause constipation.

*IRON*

Iron is important for the production of hemoglobin, which transports oxygen to your cells. It also supports oxygen in your muscles and helps your immune system.

**Why is it important?** The volume of blood in your body increases by up to 50 percent during pregnancy, and your body will need iron in order to create hemoglobin to match this increase. Your baby and placenta also needs iron to develop. Iron deficiency is linked to preterm delivery, low birth weight and infant mortality.

**Examples of food**: Red meat, poultry, fish, kidney beans, oatmeal, chickpeas, spinach, bread, raisins

**Consumption suggestions**: Cook in an iron-cast pan or skillet, as moist and acidic foods such as tomato sauce soak up iron. Make sure to include a lot of iron-rich foods in your diet and ask your doctor about supplements.

*FOLIC ACID*

Folic acid, folates or vitamin B9 as it is also called, is recommended to all women of childbearing age due to its importance during pregnancy.

**Why is it important?** Folic acid helps prevent neural tube defects, defects of the spinal cord and the brain. These defects occur in the earliest stages of pregnancy, and women trying to conceive should therefore always take folic acid supplements to reduce the risk.

**Examples of food**: Lentils, beans, asparagus, broccoli, spinach, edamame beans, citrus fruit and juice.

**Consumption suggestions**: Prepare for yourself daily a salad that consists of green vegetables that have a high value of folic acid. Use as a base for these salads fresh spinach. If you don't eat enough food that contains folic acid you should consult with your doctor about taking folic acid supplements.

*ZINC*

Your body always needs zinc for producing, maintaining and repairing DNA as well as building cells.

**Why is it important?** Zinc is vital for the fast growth of cells during pregnancy. It helps boost your immune system and also helps wounds heal faster. Zinc deficiency has been linked to miscarriage, low birth weight and toxemia.

**Examples of food**: Cereals, red meat, poultry, beans, nuts, whole grains and yogurt.

**Consumption suggestions**: Make sure you eat enough food that contains zinc,. If you do not, you should consult your doctor about taking prenatal vitamins that include the zinc you need. It is better to eat foods originating from animals such as turkey and red meat since they absorb the zinc better in the body. If you're vegetarian, it's important to consume the zinc separately, from dairy products and calcium supplements, for an effective absorption. There is a number of ways of processing food that contributes to the absorption of zinc: sprouting or soaking the beans, seeds, nuts and grains. whole meal bread leavening and eating roasted nuts.

## MAGNESIUM

Magnesium is a chemical element and an alkaline earth metal.

**Why is it important?** Magnesium helps build and repair tissue. It also aids in the building of bones and teeth. Deficiency can lead to preeclampsia, decreased fetal growth and mortality. A good amount of magnesium can keep contractions from occurring prematurely.

**Examples of food**: Whole grains, salmon, sunflower seeds, spaghetti, soybeans, potatoes, bananas

**Consumption suggestions**: Eat salads that contain green vegetables. Sprinkle sunflower seeds, almonds and cashew nuts on top for a varied diet. If you haven't been able to eat much due to morning sickness, talk to your doctor about taking a supplement.

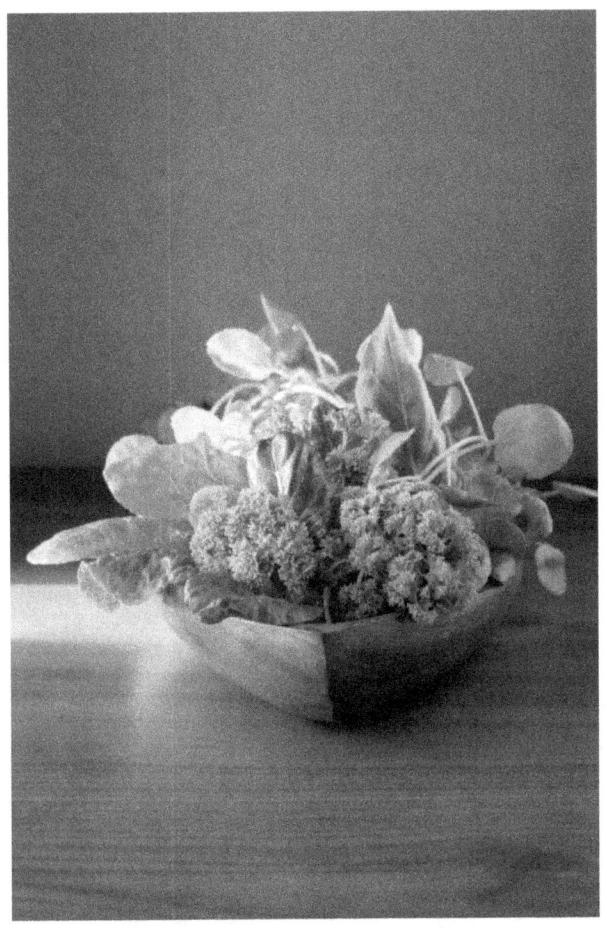

*CHROMIUM*

Chromium is a chemical element with a steely, lustrous color.

**Why is it important?** Chromium helps break down and store fats, carbohydrates and proteins. It also helps maintain normal levels of blood sugar together with insulin. It aids the building of proteins in your baby's body.

**Examples of food**: Cheese, peanut butter, spinach, chicken, apples, broccoli.

**Consumption suggestions**: Include chromium-rich foods in your diet.

*WATER*

Remember to drink plenty of fluids, especially water, during your pregnancy. Water carries nutrients to your baby and helps prevent dehydration. It can help you avoid constipation, hemorrhoids and bladder infections. You will need plenty of water to support the increased amount of blood in your system.

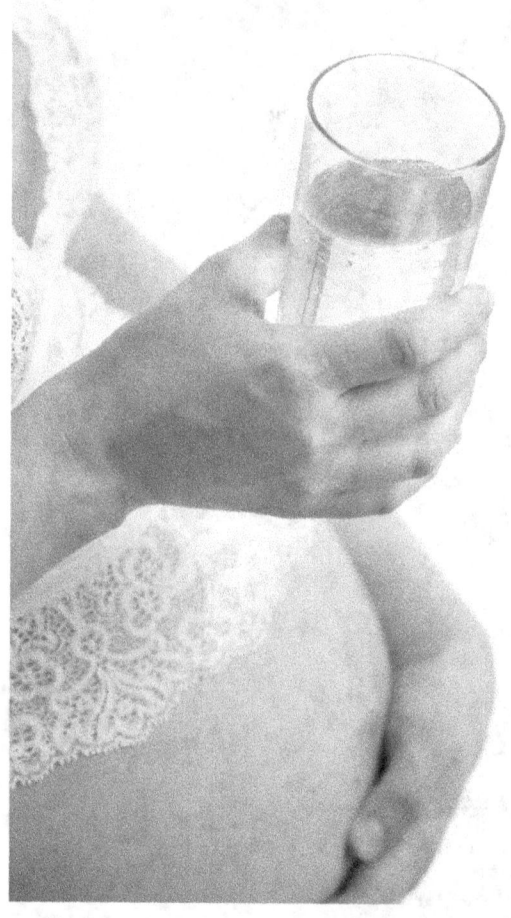

Knowing what nutrients are needed for you and your baby is an important step, but it's also important to know what you should avoid. This is something we will look at in the next chapter in the book.

*"He who takes medicine and neglects his diet wastes the skills of his doctors."*

*~ Chinese proverb*

# Chapter 5- What should you avoid ingesting during pregnancy?

In the last chapter, we talked about what kinds of ingredients you should eat, but there are some **you should avoid when pregnant**. The reason is that some types of food can contain bacteria, and other substances that are harmful to your baby.

◎ ◎ ◎ ◎ ◎ ◎ ◎

*Elizabeth hadn´t read about food safety while pregnant with her first child, and as a lover of sushi she often ate raw fish. Normally this would not have put her at risk, but with a child developing in her uterus she was now no longer only eating for herself. In her second trimester she had food poisoning and was forced to seek medical attention. Her doctors did a wonderful job, and luckily her child was not hurt by the incident. They did warn her about the dangers of raw food, however, and she stayed away from raw fish until after the birth of a healthy daughter.*

◎ ◎ ◎ ◎ ◎ ◎ ◎

It's important to know about the risks involved with the consumption of certain types of food so that you can avoid them while pregnant. In this chapter, we will look at what kinds of food to stay away from and why.

### Alcohol

Doctors are not entirely sure what the effects are of drinking alcohol while pregnant, and it is therefore recommended to stay away from it. Alcohol reaches your baby through the placenta. Heavy drinking can seriously harm your baby´s development and cause FASD (Fetal Alcohol Spectrum Disorder). A study has also shown that even moderate drinking of one or two glasses of wine per week can harm your baby´s IQ.

### Artificial Sweeteners

Artificial sweeteners contain a lot of empty calories which are added  to the diet but which do not contain many, if any at all, vitamins or minerals. Consumed in moderation, they are considered safe during pregnancy, but they could contribute to excessive weight gain. You might also be missing out on important vitamins if you consume a lot of diet soda instead of fruit juice, for example. Diet soda contains saccharin, which is a sweetener considered unsafe during pregnancy, since it is proven to cross the placenta and can remain in the baby's tissue.

## Saturated fats and trans fats

Unhealthy fats such as saturated fats and trans fats should be avoided as much as possible during pregnancy since they can build up cholesterol and fat stores in your body. Studies have linked trans fats to an increased risk of heart attacks, cancer and diabetes. There is also some evidence linking trans fats to low birth weights. Try to replace your cooking oils with unsaturated fats like safflower oil and avoid fatty meat or deep-fried food.

## Refined white flour and sugar products

Carbohydrates such as sugar and items baked with white flour contain the so-called "bad" carbohydrates because they do not provide the necessary substitutes for an adequate nutrition to your body. They can cause extreme fluctuations in the sugar levels in your blood. They come at the expense of "good" carbohydrates, which can lead to overeating. When you surrender to your desires (cakes, ice cream, etc.) you prevent your body getting the nutritions it demands. "Good" carbohydrates can be found in whole grains and legumes .

## Caffeine

Many studies have found a link between high caffeine intake and miscarriages or stillbirths. Caffeine is a stimulant that raises your heart rate and can cause insomnia and heartburn. Your baby cannot process the caffeine they receive from the placenta and could therefore be hurt by it. Coffee and tea, which are the most common sources of caffeine, also contain compounds which make it harder for the body to absorb iron. Consider switching to decaffeinated coffee, which contains only small amounts of caffeine, and stick to 200 mg of caffeine a day.

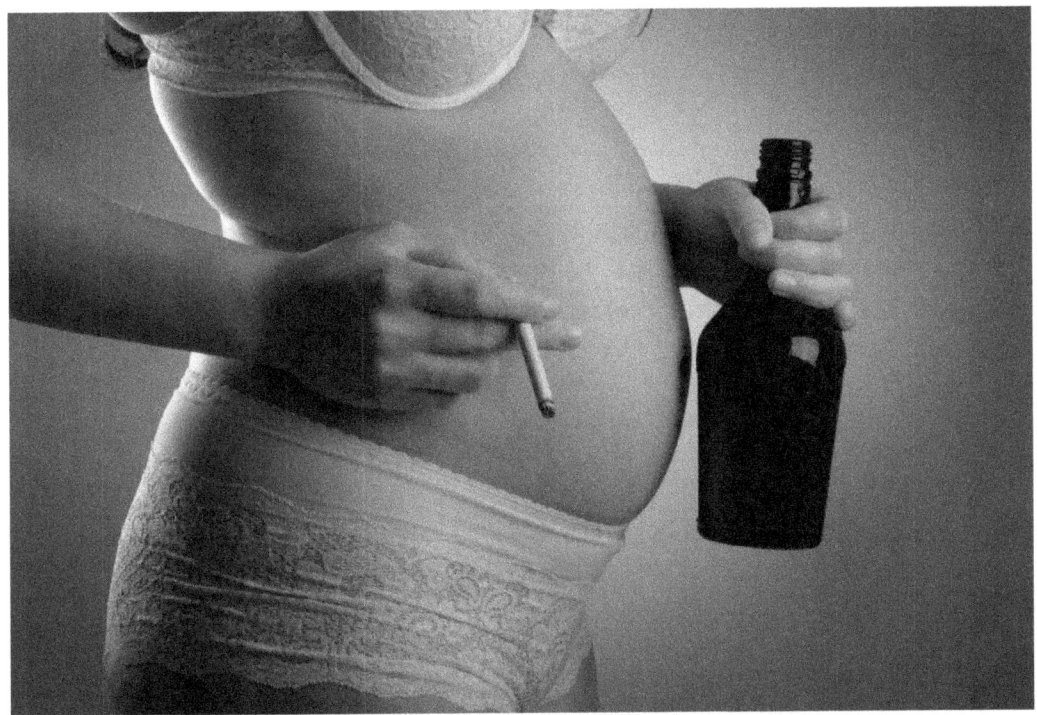

### Salt and monosodium glutamate (MSG)

Salt can raise blood pressure, but it is considered safe to consume in moderate quantities during your pregnancy. If you have no trouble with MSG before your pregnancy, it can be consumed in moderate amounts.

### Fish

Oily fish is good for you, but fish and seafood can contain environmental pollutants that can harm your baby. It is therefore recommended that you limit your intake to no more than two portions of fish a week. Swordfish, shark and marlin contain unsafe amounts of mercury that can harm your baby. Tuna contains mercury as well, so make sure not to eat too much of it. You should not eat raw fish or seafood during your pregnancy since they can cause food poisoning.

### Partially cooked meat, poultry and eggs

Eggs, meat and poultry may contain salmonella bacteria which can cause a serious illness potentially harmful to your growing baby. Make sure all your meals containing these ingredients are well cooked. Avoid products which may contain unpasteurized eggs such as restaurant- or self-made mousse, ice cream and mayonnaise. Products from the supermarket, however, such as dressings or mayonnaise, are usually safe since they contain pasteurized eggs.

### Soft cheeses

You should avoid soft and mould-ripened cheeses like Brie, Camembert and Chevre during your pregnancy. The same goes for soft and blue-veined cheeses like Roquefort and Gorgonzola. You can, however, eat them if they have been heated all the way through. These cheeses can contain Listeria which causes listeriosis, an illness with flu-like symptoms that can severely harm your baby and even cause a miscarriage.

### Unpasteurized juice and dairy products

Unpasteurized milk, products made with unpasteurized milk and fruit juices can contain bacteria that can cause food poisoning, so avoid them during your pregnancy. Food poisoning is linked to E. Coli and salmonella which can make you very ill and potentially harm your child.

### Sprouts

Raw sprouts are very nutritious, but they also contain bacteria that can be harmful to your baby. Make sure to cook all your sprouts before eating them.

### Peanuts

Eating peanuts or peanut butter increases the risk of your child developing peanut allergies. You are more likely to increase the risk during your third trimester, so it's a good idea to limit peanut consumption during this time and while breastfeeding.

### Herbal tea

Many herbs used in herbal teas are not harmful in low quantities, but when concentrated in tea they can be harmful to your child. Some have even been linked to an increased risk of miscarriage, early labor and low birth weight. Raspberry tea can, for example, be used to aid delivery but may cause preterm labor.

### Sweets

Try replacing sweets with natural products such as dates extract and almond butter. A combination of tahini and honey will have the same taste as halvah, and dry fruits are healthy snacks, without unhealthy sugar.

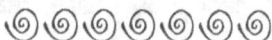

*Mary drank a lot of diet soda before she found out that she was pregnant. It was important for her to not drink a lot of sugar in order not to gain extra pounds. When she learned of the negative effects of artificial sweeteners and how they could harm her baby, she switched to freshly pressed juices and water. Since she kept a healthy diet, she didn't gain weight like she feared she would,  and felt healthier than ever when  her baby boy was born.*

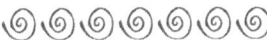

As long as you eat cautiously and remain aware of what foods could be harmful to your baby, you should remain at low risk from bacteria. **Remember to eat sensibly and take everything in moderation.**

Now that you know about the foods that are good for you, and about those that can harm you, it's time to take action. In the next chapter we'll plan your daily menu that will be based on all the foods we discussed in the previous chapters.

*"One should eat to live, not live to eat."*

*~ Moliere (French playwright and actor )*

# CHAPTER 6- HOW TO PLAN YOUR WEEKLY MENU

## THE IMPORTANCE OF PLANNING AHEAD

Now that you've been working on the mental side of eating healthy and have learned what foods you should and shouldn't eat, you can take steps to begin eating healthy.

A simple and effective way to ensure that you go through with your new plan is to make a weekly menu packed with healthy meals. This will reduce stress, both in the supermarket and at home when the time has come to begin cooking.

**A lack of planning usually leads us to eat what is available: Processed foods, snacks, fast food and other meals that are unhealthy, especially during your pregnancy. Some of these foods may even contain ingredients from the previous chapter which could harm both you and your child.**

French-fries and certain chips often contain trans fats, which build up your cholesterol and increases the risk of heart attacks and diabetes. Ice cream, sweets and soda contain sugar while diet soda contains artificial sweeteners. Processed foods and fast food often contain additives and a lot of salt, all of which when consumed excessively, could harm both you and your child.

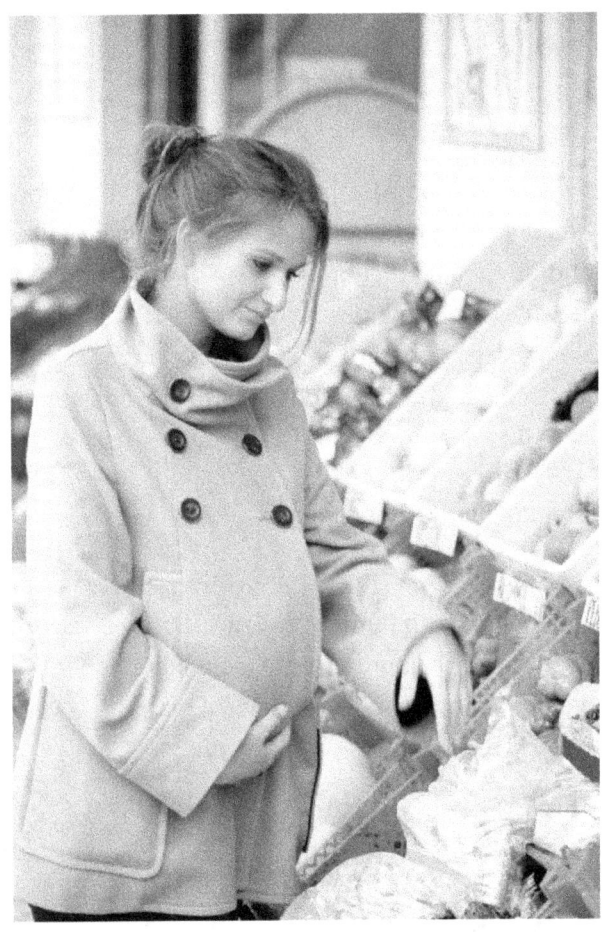

◎ ◎ ◎ ◎ ◎ ◎ ◎

*Mary-Anne had read up on healthy food during her pregnancy and fully intended to eat healthy. Most of her life she had been eating fast food and ready-meals due to a stressful job and a tight schedule, but with a baby on the way she wanted to make a change for both of their sakes.*

*She had prepared a vision board and found a few recipes that would help her. What she had not done was plan ahead. Every week, she'd find out she had nothing healthy in the fridge and no ideas on what to cook. Her busy life prevented her from spending a lot of time in the supermarket and eventually she'd end up buying pizzas and burgers for dinner. Even though her doctors warned her, she never seemed able to make a change.*

*Her daughter was born healthy despite Mary-Anne's diet, but she was at a risk of developing diabetes. Mary-Anne was more determined than ever to change their diets and make sure her daughter ate healthy throughout her childhood. Now, she began planning a week ahead and found the method to be more effective than she could ever have imagined.*

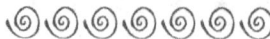

Planning ahead is an important component in your success to eat foods that are nutritious for you and your baby. It will ensure that you only have healthy food available and lessen the temptation for a late-night ice cream or a pizza dinner. Instead of chips for snacks you will now have nuts and popcorn; instead of ready-meals you will have meals that are quick and easy to prepare and at the same time nutritious. It will help you stay on a balanced and healthy diet good for both you and your baby.

## PLANNING AHEAD: PRACTICAL STEPS
When planning your menu, do the following:

**Step 1:**
List all the foods that contain a high nutritional value. Use previous chapters in this book and combine the knowledge with your personal taste. Remember that you should aim for a good balance between meals and eat nothing in excess.

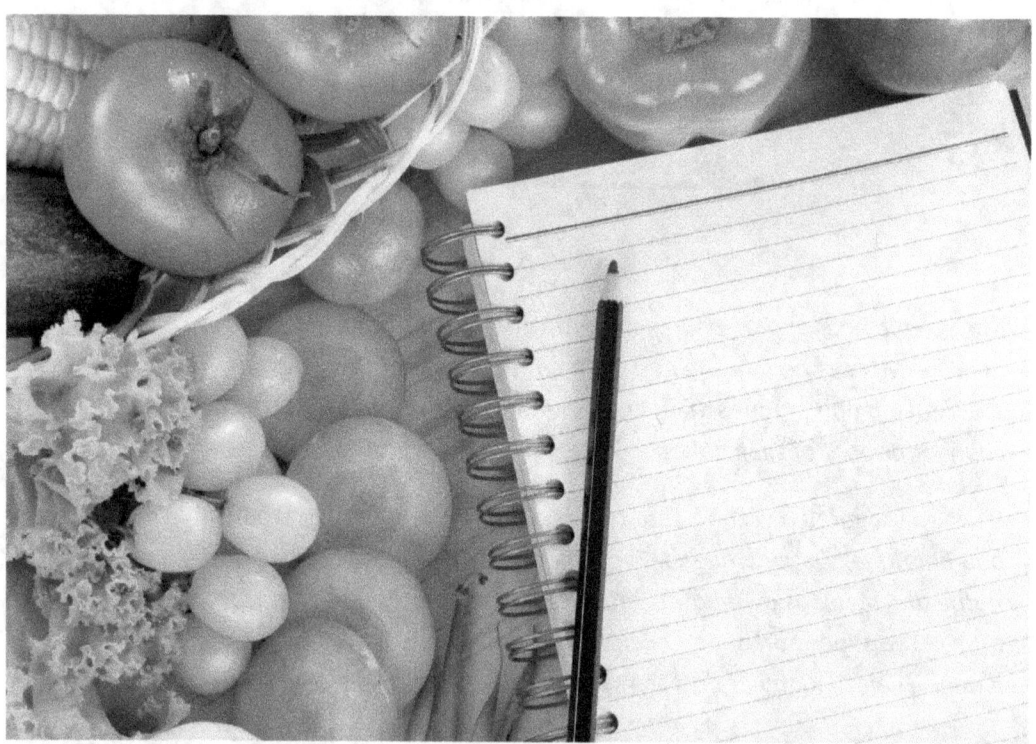

**Step 2:**

Fill in the following table with meals that you like and that provide you with the necessary nutrients.

| Meal | Sunday | Monday | Tuesday | Wednesday | Thursday | Friday | Saturday |
|------|--------|--------|---------|-----------|----------|--------|----------|
| Breakfast | | | | | | | |
| Snack | | | | | | | |
| Lunch | | | | | | | |
| Afternoon snack | | | | | | | |
| Dinner | | | | | | | |
| Bedtime snack* | | | | | | | |

*Some women might skip this last meal since it can make it harder to fall sleep. If you have trouble sleeping, leave this one out.

You can find ideas for *simple daily menus* if you scan the following code:

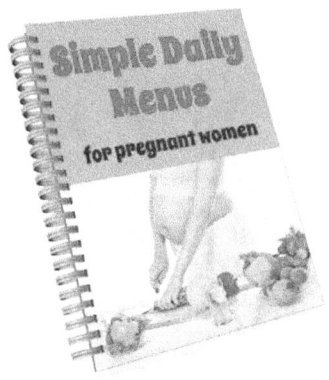

**Step 3:**

Once you have the table filled out, create your menu for the following week. Choose combinations that suit your taste and that fulfill your criteria of cooking time/simplicity as well as nutrients. Prepare a shopping list. You are always free to plan ahead as far as you like and choose the frequency of the food shopping. If planning for two weeks ahead suits you, go ahead and do so.

**Step 4:**

Once a week (or any frequency you've chosen) go to the supermarket and buy the food on your list. Be ready to stick to your list in the supermarket instead of giving in to urges for sweets, chips or other unhealthy foods.

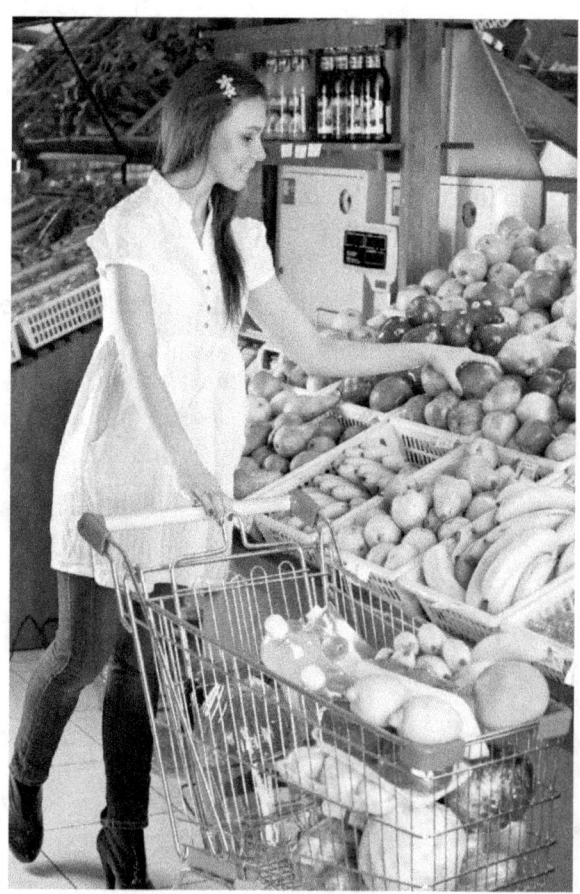

**Step 5:**

Now it is time to prepare the food. This can be the breaking point for you if you don't like to spend much time in the kitchen. But since you have come all this way, don't give up just yet. In the next chapter we will look at how to prepare meals quickly and easily without hassle.

You are now on your way to a nourishing and a healthy diet.

In the next chapter I'll introduce you to an easy method for preparing the wonderful menu you created.

IMPORTANT POINTS TO CONSIDER

- Even when you have menus planned it is okay to deviate for special events or situations. Don't feel stressed about having to stick to this schedule on a day where for some reason it doesn't suit you. All the other regular meals will provide you with nutrients enough to make one day's deviation insignificant to your or your child's well-being.
- If you buy food in your workplace, plan accordingly. Stay aware of what you should and shouldn't eat at a diner or food stand.
- If you have a family, they will also enjoy the benefits of eating healthy and nutritious food. By making these menus and sticking to them, you are caring not only for yourself and your baby but for the rest of the family as well.

*Angelina had a stressful job where she rarely had time for lunch and felt she had no time left over for cooking. Her husband's schedule was similar. When she got pregnant with their first child, she decided she wanted to make a change. She set up a weekly menu and used Seinfeld's method of persistence from chapter 4 in this book to encourage her to go through with it. Every day she and her husband ate healthy, they marked a cross on the calendar. They resisted the urges to buy ready-meals or go out to restaurants and learned to cook simple and healthy meals for both of them.*

*Eventually they began to feel they had more energy and more time to themselves even though they spent more time in the kitchen. Angelina's husband became involved in the menu and they found out they actually liked cooking. When their son was born they continued eating healthy food and felt full of energy even as parents to a newborn.*

*"By failing to prepare, you are preparing to fail."*

*~ Benjamin Franklin (Author, Politician, Scientist, and Inventor)*

# CHAPTER 7- AN IDEA FOR EASILY PREPARING NUTRITIOUS FOOD FOR BUSY PREGNANT WOMEN

## WHAT ARE THE FACTORS THAT HINDER YOU?

Now that you have prepared your weekly menu and done the shopping, you should be ready to spend some time in the kitchen. Many women associate healthy food with lengthy preparation times, complicated recipes and plenty of effort. This can cause them to give up on eating healthy and continue with their current eating habits.

There are also women who wouldn't want to spend a lot of time in the kitchen cooking healthy food. Many have stressful jobs and lots to do in their spare time other than preparing a meal. Some don't believe that they can cook.

It doesn't have to be that way. Healthy food does not have to take longer than unhealthy food and it can be very easy to cook.

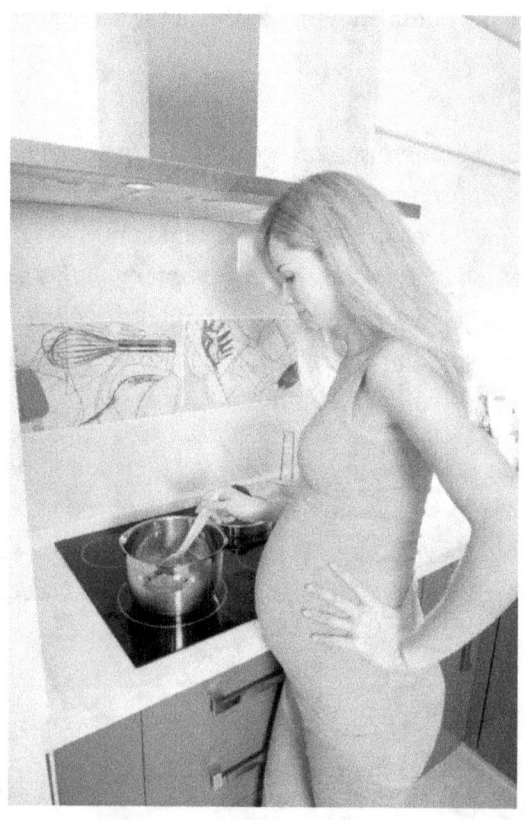

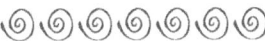

*Jasmine had problems with her weight her whole life, and knew she should blame it on the ready-meals and fast food she was eating. Her stressful job as well as a busy evening schedule prevented her from ever spending much time in the kitchen. When she found out she was pregnant, she was told she should change her habits and de-stress, or both she and her baby could suffer.*

*Jasmine thought cooking healthy meals was an impossible task that she would never be able to pull off. She believed she would only be able to find healthy meals that she wouldn't enjoy eating and that she would never be able to cook them. She stuck to her old habits of eating fast food instead.*

*Halfway through her pregnancy however, her doctor warned that her blood pressure was too high and that she was at a risk of developing diabetes. Even if the baby would be safe, Jasmine might not be. This warning triggered in her husband a desire to learn about cooking. He eventually taught her how she could make simple but healthy meals. Jasmine's blood pressure went down and she didn't gain any unnecessary weight during her pregnancy thanks to her improved diet.*

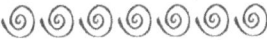

**You have come all this way through the book, so don't give up! Remember that preparing and cooking healthy food can be easy as well as fast if you follow a few simple guidelines.**

THE EASY SOLUTION FOR PREPARING HEALTHY FOOD

**The solution to long cooking times and hard work is what I call** Concentrated Effort. Instead of spending a lot of time in the kitchen every day, focus your meal preparation efforts on one day every week or so. You can decide for yourself what works best for you. During this one day you could prepare a number of dishes together, enabling you to cook quickly and easily during the rest of the week.

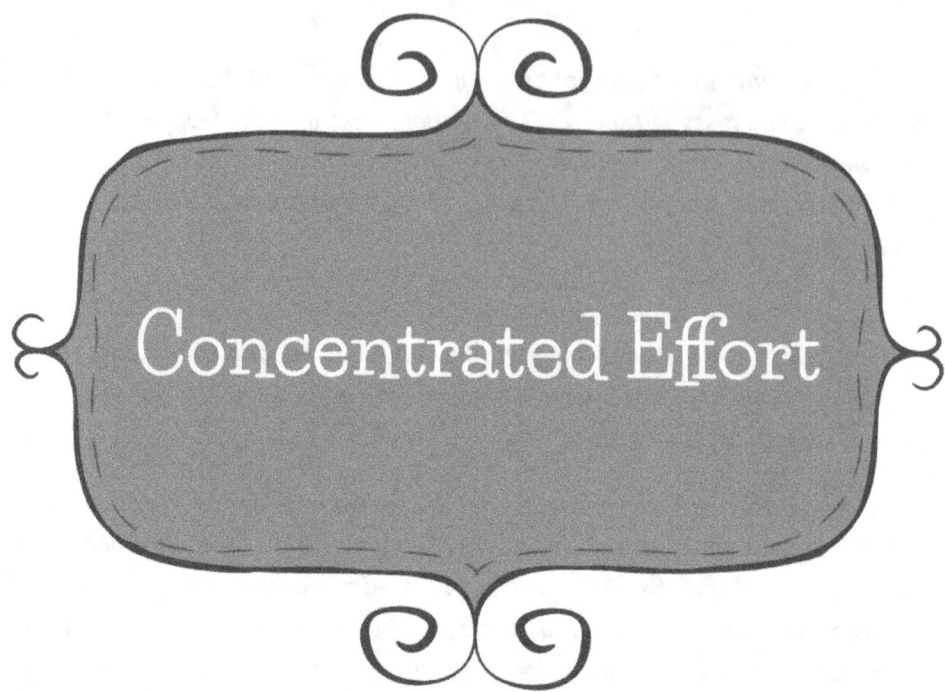

# Concentrated Effort

When you prepare a number of dishes at the same time, you utilize your resources as well as your time spent in the kitchen. Instead of digging up recipes or trying to find ingredients, you have everything ready at this one day. By doing this, you can save hours of cooking time and make sure that you cook only when you have a lot of time available for cooking. All your meals will be easy to heat up during your week and you will find it much easier to stick to a healthy diet.

**Here is what you do to prepare your meals efficiently, once a week or less often if you want to.**

1.  Make sure you have plenty of space in the freezer and Tupperware for convenient storage during the week. If you don't have these handy containers, make sure to buy some in various sizes and think of a way to mark them clearly so you will know which meal belongs to which day. I recommend arranging the containers by the type of meal (lunch, dinner, etc.), so that they will be easy to find and reheat.

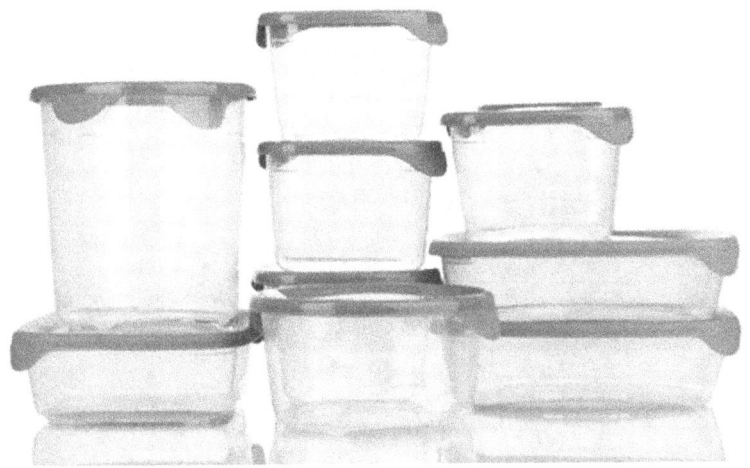

2. Pick a day of the week when you will do the cooking. Set some time aside during this day. From my experience, you will need about one to two hours, but be prepared to give it more time if you have a time-consuming meal and/or limited space on your stove.

3. Take the weekly menu and check which meals can be prepared in advance. Remember that some meals can lose a lot of nutrition when reheated and that salads, etc., can have short expiration dates.

4. Make sure that you have the necessary ingredients available in your house. Plan ahead so that you do your grocery shopping just before it's time to cook if you intend to buy fresh vegetables or raw meat.

5. Place in the freezer those meals you don't need right away and defrost them during the week. This will make bringing lunch to work easy as well, since you'll already have the meals ready.

6. Put on some good music, roll up your sleeves and get cooking. For each week, the cooking will become easier and less of a chore. You will notice how it becomes a habit to have one day of cooking each week, and soon you will discover how much time you can save and how the healthy food affects your energy levels.

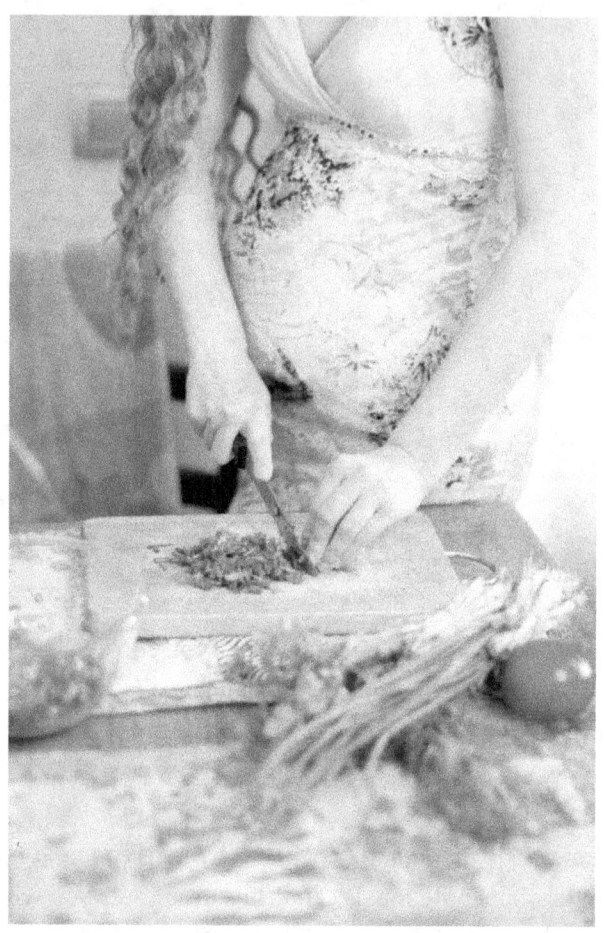

7.  It is important that you keep your weekly menu visible to you on the refrigerator door or elsewhere in the kitchen so that you always stick to the menu. Remember that persistence is important and that you are now building a good habit.

8.  Don't forget to give yourself positive reinforcements. Celebrate your success of eating healthy every week with a special treat. If you have been eating expensive restaurant meals before, why not take the money you'll be saving by cooking at home and treat yourself to something special? Or allow yourself to have your favorite snack when you've finished a week of healthy eating.

9.  When you're done with the weekly cooking, take a step back and appreciate what you have accomplished. In a few hours you have prepared healthy and nutritious food for the whole week.

10. Now all that is left is to start eating!

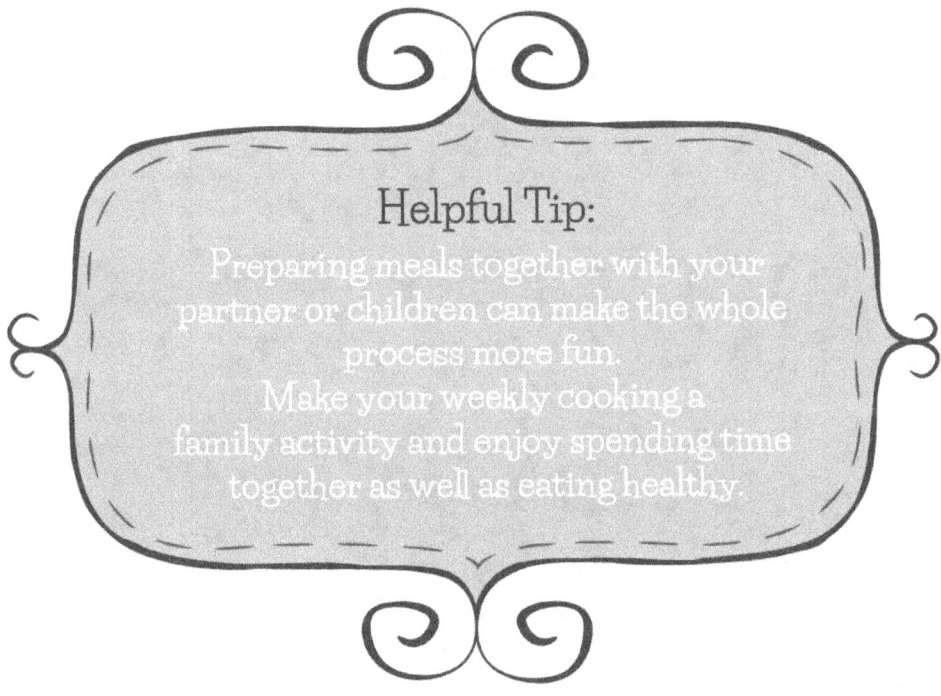

*Rosie had gone back to school when she was pregnant with her second child. Her son was uninterested in eating healthy during her pregnancy and her husband was as bad as she was at cooking. Instead of giving up and resorting to fast food, however, Rosie set up a weekly schedule and made the whole family pitch in. Eventually it became a habit and she had healthy food throughout her pregnancy and a long time afterwards.*

*"Never consider the possibility of failure; as long as you persist, you will be successful."*

*~ Brian Tracy (motivational speaker and author)*

Helpful Tip:
Preparing meals together with your partner or children can make the whole process more fun.
Make your weekly cooking a family activity and enjoy spending time together as well as eating healthy.

# CHAPTER 8- FOOD PREPARATION SHORTCUTS FOR SUPER-BUSY PREGNANT WOMEN

You now know that eating healthy is important for you, but you may still find the instructions in the previous chapters hard to follow. It can seem like cooking takes forever and that you never manage to stick to the menu.

**Don't worry, I have more tricks that I want to share with you.**

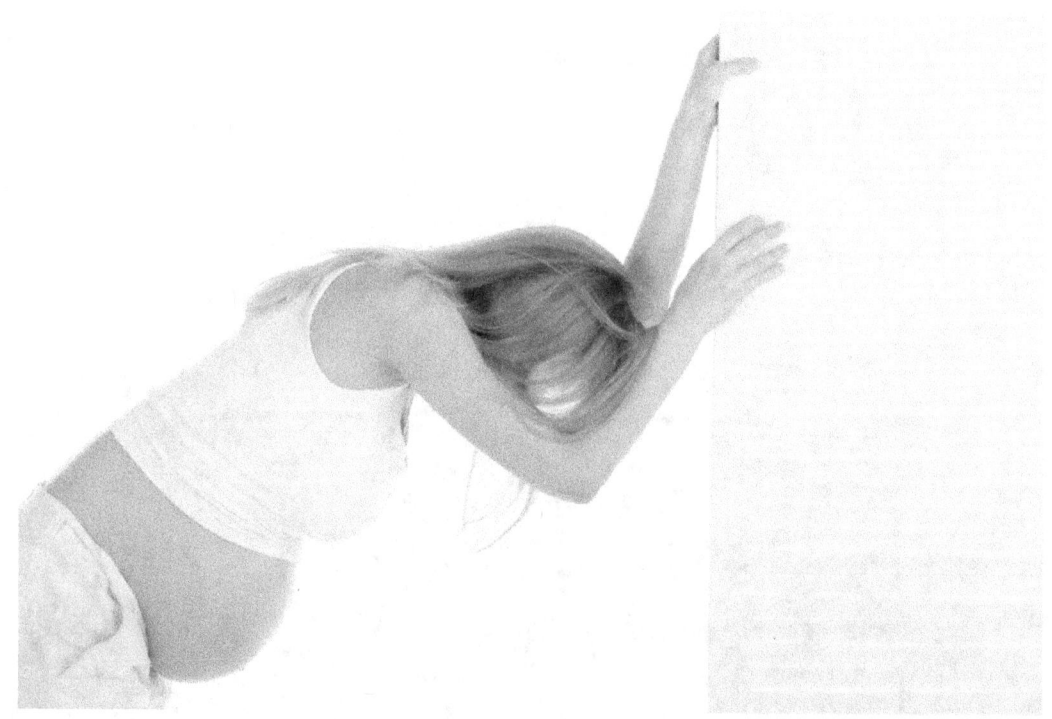

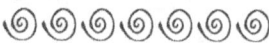

*Eleanor felt she couldn't master cooking no matter how hard she tried. Even with a weekly schedule and cooking only once a week, she felt meal preparation times took too long. She also kept returning to ready-meals simply because she didn't feel like eating what she had already prepared and placed in her freezer.*

*Eventually she gave up and returned to eating unhealthy fast food and ready-meals. Her blood pressure increased and her doctors warned her of the high content of fat and salt in the food she was eating. They also advised her to at least eat some nutritious meals so that the baby would get the vitamins and minerals he needed for healthy growth.*

*Eleanor ignored their advice, since she felt she had done what she could already. Her daughter was born underweight, and Eleanor wondered if she would be able to give her the necessary nutrients through the breast milk. Eleanor had always wanted to breastfeed her baby and decided it was time to make a change. Now she gave herself some room to eat what she wanted but decided to make at least one meal a day a healthy one. Eventually her daughter gained weight and received the nutrients she needed.*

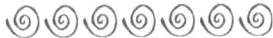

In order to find out why you're having trouble sticking to your weekly menu, try to think about what it is that makes you fail. Don't judge yourself too harshly at this point, but try to remain positive and intent on succeeding.

## SUPER-EASY SOLUTIONS FOR SUPER-BUSY WOMEN

There are still a few other options available to you if you find it too hard to stick to eating healthy at this point. Which one you choose is up to you, and the only wrong decision you can make here is to give up and return to your old eating habits.

One solution is to hire the services of a cook. This might require a large monetary expense but it will save you time and effort. When calculating the cost, you should also include the total amount you spent on food before you decided to eat healthy. If you ate out often , a cook might cost only a little more or the same as all those meals at a restaurant (including transportation there and back).

The other solution is to use the shortcuts which I'm about to give you in this chapter. You can combine these recommendations with cooking some good meals throughout the week.

The third solution is to combine the two above and hire a cook's service for some of the time. Then, on other days, use the following shortcuts for preparing meals on your own.

If you do decide to utilize the services of a cook, make sure that he or she is aware of the nutrition recommendations in the previous chapters. Not all cooks are used to cooking meals for pregnant women so you might want to ensure that you'll be getting the nutrition you and your baby require.

## EASY SHORTCUTS EVERY SUPER-BUSY WOMAN CAN USE

The following shortcuts will help you cut time from lengthy meal preparation.

Sandwiches

A sandwich with whole-wheat bread without additives can provide a healthy and filling snack or even a full meal. Spread  hummus or avocado on your sandwich  to add health benefits. Add vegetables, cold turkey and  other healthy ingredients you like. Sandwiches are easy to prepare, they can be  ready in no time and can be suited to your personal taste.

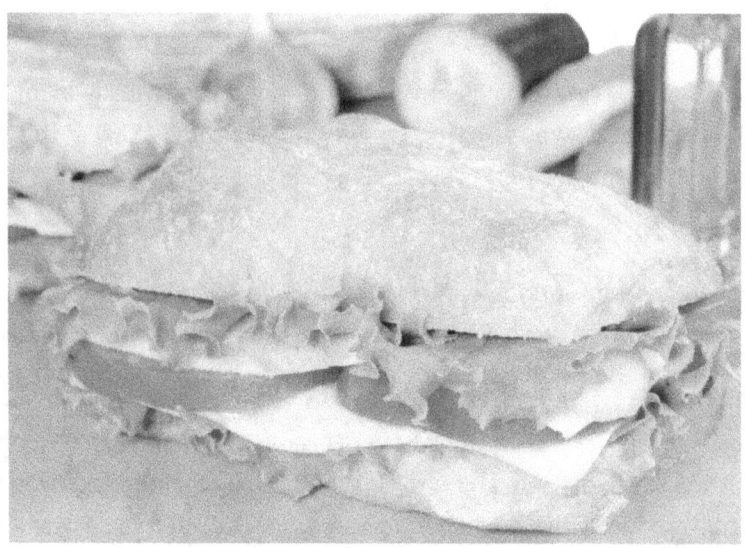

Dried fruit

Women on the go can benefit from bringing some dried fruit with them, to eat between meals. This will provide you with important nutrients and fill you up effectively at the same time. Make sure to buy dry organic fruit in order to avoid sulfuric acid.

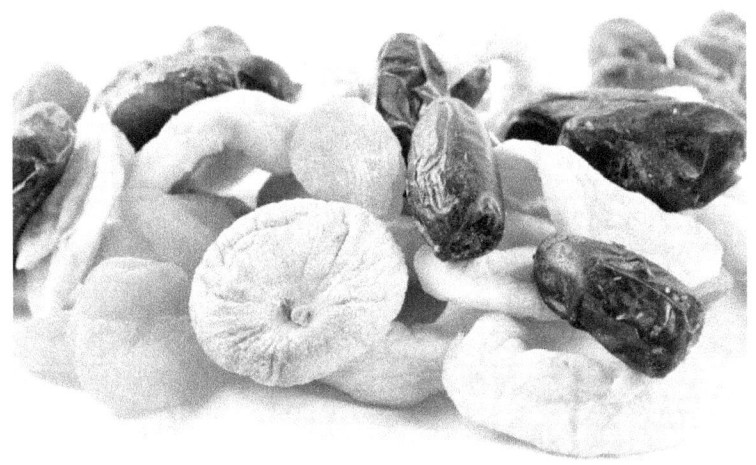

Bowl of cereal

Eat a bowl of whole-grain cereal as a full meal. Whole-grain cereals are healthy and will fill you up effectively. Don't add any sugar as this is an empty carbohydrate without any health benefits.

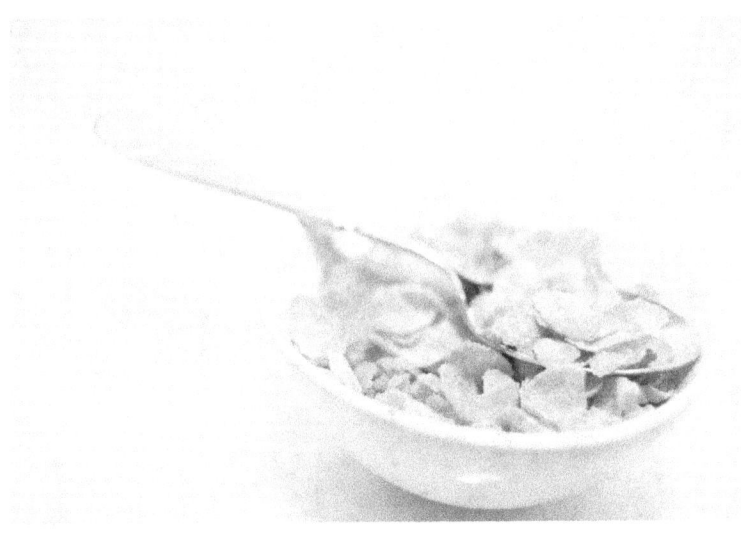

Soup

If you don't feel like cutting up vegetables, buy a bag of frozen vegetables and put them in a soup. This is a healthy and filling meal without requiring much time or effort.

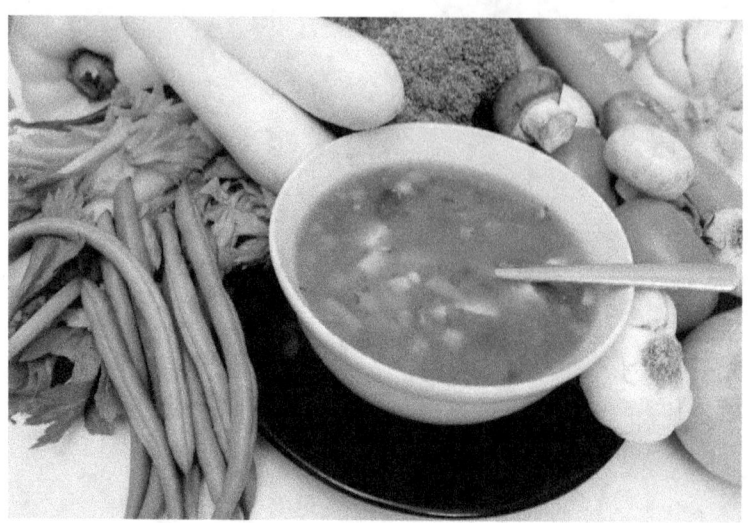

Buy vegetables in all colors and cut them up at the same time. Put them in a Tupperware container and keep it handy when you need a snack or when you want to add a healthy salad to your meal.

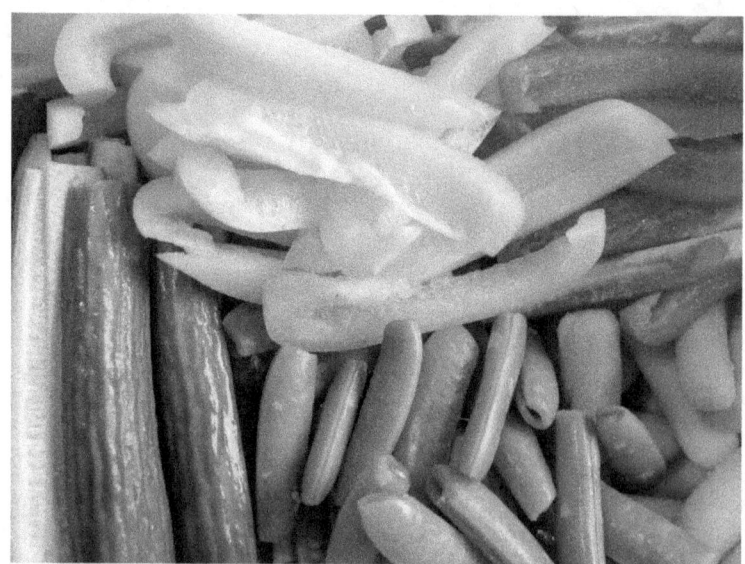

Fruit

Eat plenty of fruit, which will keep you going throughout the day. Not only are they packed with healthy vitamins, they are filling and easy to bring anywhere you go. Choose fruit that require peeling or make sure you wash the fruit before eating it.

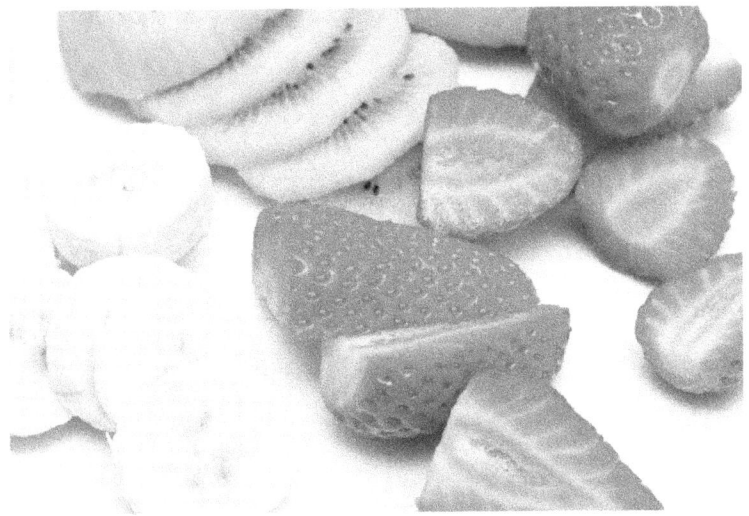

### Eggs

Prepare a pot of boiled eggs and eat an egg every day. Eggs are very filling and packed with proteins and nutrition. They are easy to eat alone or can be added to any meal to give it a healthy twist.

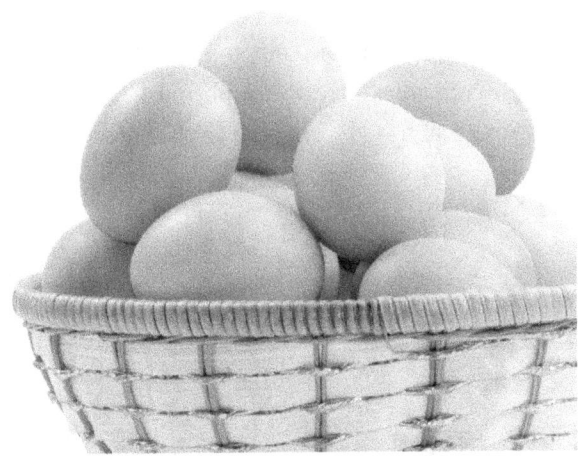

### Fruit or vegetable shake/smoothie

Fruits and vegetables contain a lot of vitamins and nutrients that you can consume in a tasty and simple way. Make a smoothie from your own favorite fruits; this will also help prepare you in making healthy smoothies when the baby has arrived. Drink it together with a meal to add some nutrients or alone as a healthy snack.

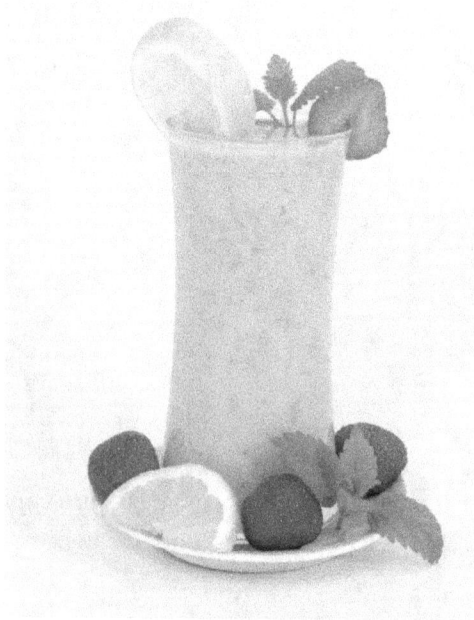

### Chicken

Chicken contains a lot of protein and nutrients that are healthy for you and your baby. You can buy ready-made chicken at the supermarket and eat it together with any meal. Just remember not to buy fried chicken since that often contains unhealthy fats.

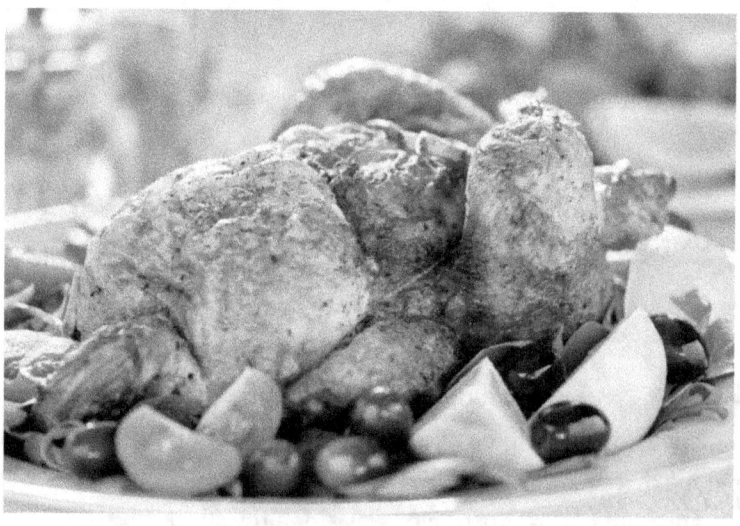

## Quaker oats

Buy Quaker Instant and add this as a healthy snack or dessert to your other meals. Whole grains will provide you with some nutrition and will keep you full for a long time.

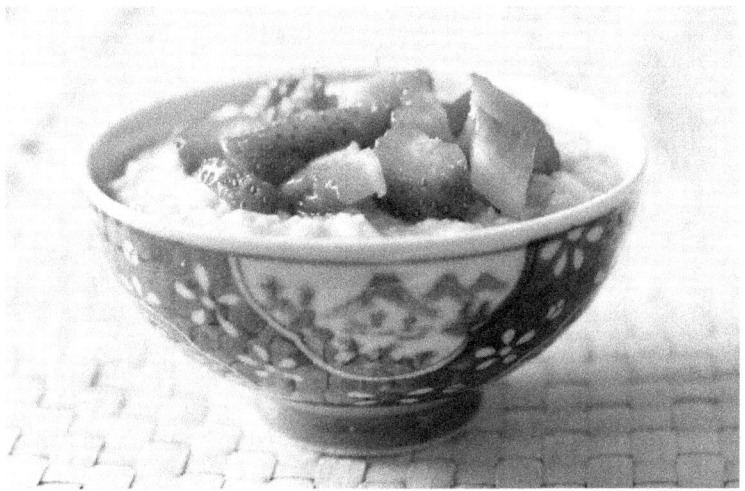

## Nuts

Nuts are healthy snacks that can be added to almost any food and eaten as a snack between meals. Choose healthy nuts such as walnuts, almonds, or sunflower seeds.

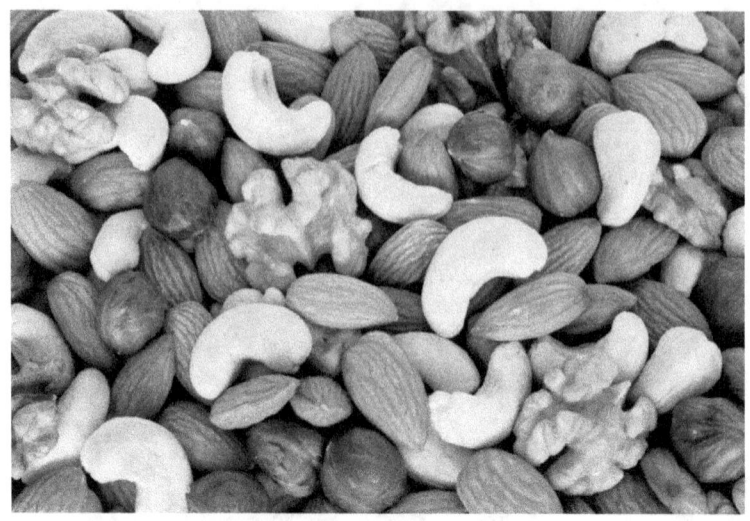

Add these foods to your diet, and you will be getting at least some of the vital nutrients for your baby. As you build a habit of eating these healthy treats, you can gradually begin to add more and more healthy meals to your daily diet.

If you still think these shortcuts seem like too much work for you, please go back to Chapter 4 and work on your mind and attitude towards eating healthy.

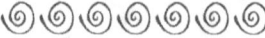

*Alice found it very difficult to eat healthy since she rarely cooked her own meals. Even cooking meals once a week felt like too much work for her. In the end she decided to give herself a break but to add a few healthy ingredients to every meal. As she ate more nuts and vegetables during the day, she found that she gained more energy than before and therefore had more time for cooking. She also developed a taste for healthy meals. At the end of her pregnancy, she was eating healthier than ever before - and enjoying it.*

*"Don't wait. The time will never be just right."*

*~ Napoleon Hill (author )*

# CHAPTER 9- FURTHER TIPS FOR HEALTHY EATING DURING PREGNANCY

By now we have looked at which types of food are recommended during your pregnancy. We have also seen which ones should be avoided during this time to help limit the risks to your growing baby. We have moved on to planning a healthy menu and preparing your healthy food with the simple "concentrated effort" method.

You've learned about the importance that your state of mind carries for this whole process and seen some tools that can help you work on that aspect. What's left now is to take action and help yourself accomplish your goal.

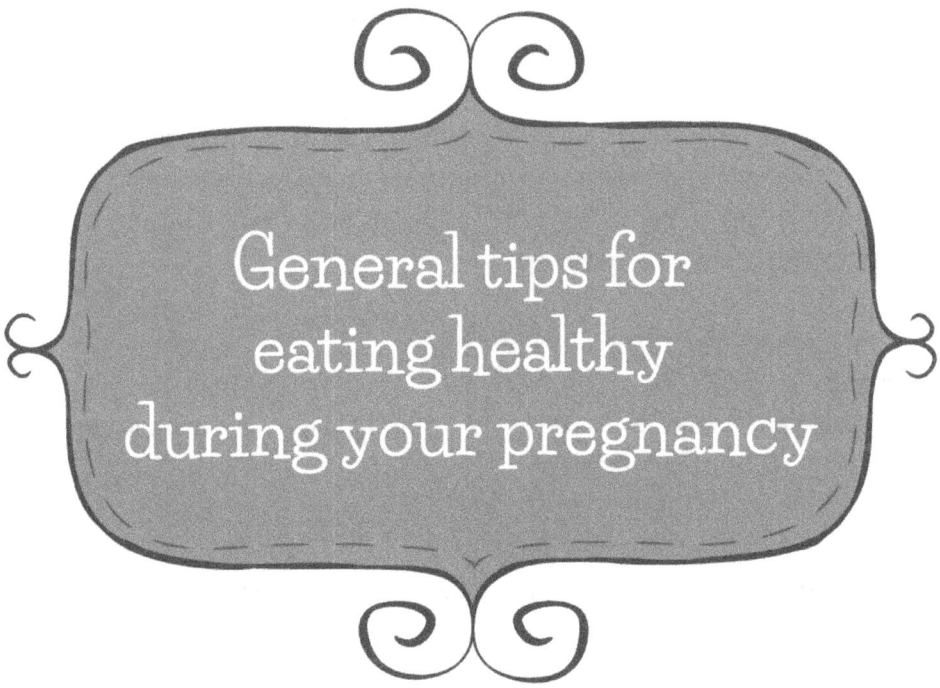

General tips for eating healthy during your pregnancy

Now we will look at some general tips for eating healthy during your pregnancy.

- Adjust the food intake level to your personal needs.
  It used to be said that a pregnant woman could "eat for two". In fact, you shouldn't eat much more at all during your pregnancy, except in the third trimester. Eating too much can add unwanted weight that can be difficult to lose afterwards, so try to limit your intake and stick to a healthy diet. Every woman is different, and how

much you eat depends on your age, physical activity, height and weight. Make sure to account for all those things when you calculate how much you should eat each day.

- **Eat a snack before bed**
  It is recommended that you eat a snack before bedtime during your pregnancy, such as a piece of fruit, yogurt or a slice of bread. This can help alleviate your nausea and let you sleep without feeling hungry.

- **Do not try any weight-loss diets during your pregnancy**
  It is recommended not to be on any diets during your pregnancy, since trying to lose weight can actually harm your baby. By trying to cut some meals from your menu, you might be robbing your growing fetus from some important nutrients. Try to see your pregnancy in a bigger perspective and use this time to develop healthy eating habits, which will help you lose weight after your baby is born.

- **Carry an Energy Kit**
  It is wise not to go too long without food during your pregnancy, since doing so can cause intense hunger or nausea. To make sure you always have a snack available, prepare an Energy Kit containing tasty snacks like nuts, fruits or yogurt, which you can carry with you wherever you go.

- **Eat small meals more often during the day**
  Eating smaller meals often rather than big and heavy meals fewer times keeps your blood sugar and energy levels stable. It can also help reduce nausea in your early pregnancy and heartburn later on.

- **Start the day with eating a handful of nuts**
  Nuts contain many healthy nutrients and will give you a tasty energy boost in the beginning of each day.

- **As long as it's not harmful, eat what you like**
  Trust in your body to tell you what foods you need. As long as it isn't harmful to you or to your baby's health, you should listen to your body and eat whatever you feel like eating. Cravings are sometimes your body's way of telling you that you need a certain type of food. Just don't overdo it and remember to eat everything in moderation.

- **Stay away from sweets and desserts**

Though they might not contain anything obviously harmful, it is not recommended to eat a lot of cake, biscuits, cookies, wafers and the like. Even if they do turn off your hunger and make you feel satisfied, they contain nothing vital for you or your baby. Instead they consist of empty calories which might cause you to gain unnecessary weight.

- Drink at least a glass of water every hour

Your body needs fluids now more than ever, in order to support your increased amount of blood as well as transport nutrients to your baby. Make sure you ingest enough liquids. Water is healthy and contains no sugars or additives, so it is a smart alternative to many other drinks out there.

- Eat home-cooked food as much as you can

Home-cooked meals contain a lot less additives and a lot more nutrients than pre-packaged food or junk food. Restaurants may be reheating their meals, causing a drop in the amount of vitamins and minerals that an ingredient contains. Cook your meals at home to make sure you get the nutrients you need.

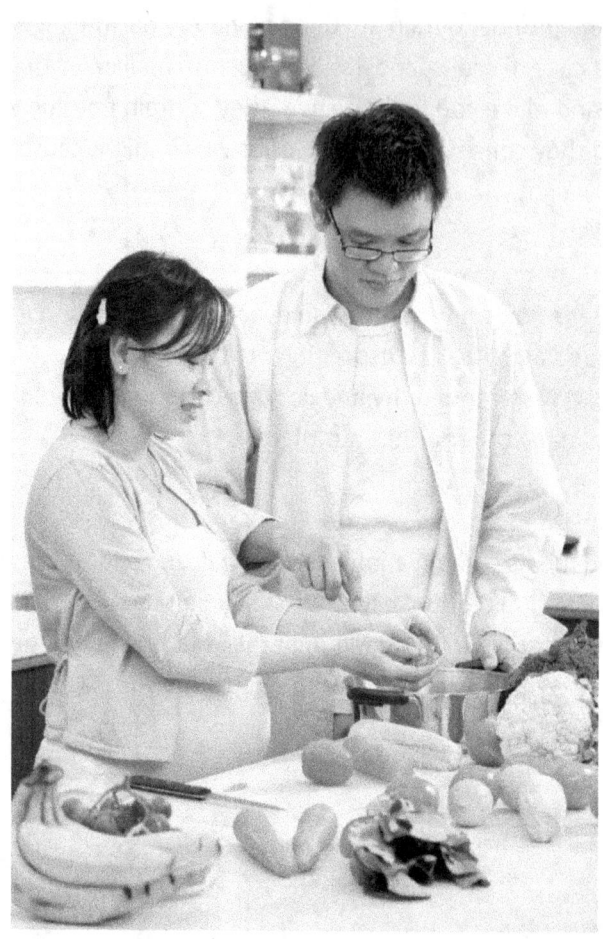

- **Pay attention to general hygiene**
  Fruits and vegetables may contain trace amounts of pesticides or bacteria. Make sure to wash them thoroughly, since you are at an increased risk of infections now that you are pregnant. Some of the bacteria on fruits or vegetables may even harm your baby.

- **Eat organic food and avoid refined products**
  Organic food will normally not contain traces of toxins or pesticides commonly found it vegetables, dairy products or meat. Refined products such as white flour, white sugar and white rice contain a lot of empty calories and may increase the risk of vaginal yeast infections.

- **Stay away from deep-fried foods**

Spare your liver from working too hard by staying away from deep-fried foods. The oil used for cooking these kinds of food is often very unhealthy and may cause you to gain excessive weight.

- Avoid animal fats

  Avoid eating animal fats and oils. These are unhealthy fats which will not benefit your baby or give you any vital nutrients. Try to switch to plant oils for cooking instead. Cold-pressed olive oil, not heated, is a particularly healthy alternative.

- Stick to your pre-pregnancy diet if it was recommended by a professional

  Some women may be on a special diet due to previous health conditions such as gestational diabetes. If that is the case, don't try to stray from your diet without consulting your doctor.

I hope these tips can come in handy when you are trying to eat healthy. Do remember that your main target is to give you and your baby the nutrients you need for a healthy development. Try not to eat anything in excess and combine a healthy diet with some form of exercise.

# CHAPTER 10- HOW TO OVERCOME COMMON PREGNANCY PROBLEMS USING A HEALTHY DIET

## COMMON PREGNANCY PROBLEMS OVERVIEW

There are many health problems that women may encounter during pregnancy. Many of these side-effects of pregnancy cause women pain, and some hinder the pregnant woman from functioning normally. A good and healthy diet with special focus on alleviating the issues that might come up can go a long way in helping you have an enjoyable pregnancy.

A pregnant woman who does not balance her diet in terms of nutrients and physical activity can have problems associated with pregnancy. The most common of these are mood swings and nausea with the latter sometimes leading to weight-loss and a lack of energy. Other problems that can occur are gestational diabetes, edema & varicose veins, anemia, lack of minerals such as calcium and zinc, imbalances of the thyroid, digestive and bowel problems, urinary tract infections and hemorrhoids. The situation can, in some of these cases become so bad, that it may affect negatively the development of the fetus.

Morning sickness can, for example, lead to fatigue and may cause you to lose those vital prenatal vitamins with minerals so important during this crucial time.

Here are some common problems you may encounter during your pregnancy and tips on what you can do to overcome them.

## NAUSEA AND VOMITING

Many pregnant women suffer from what is commonly called morning sickness, though it has nothing to do with mornings as such. The increased level of hormones in your body causes imbalances, and that in turn causes you to feel nauseous. You are most at a risk during your first trimester. Morning sickness can be reduced by taking the following precautions:

- Eat smaller meals and make sure to eat more often.
- Drink often and plenty throughout the day to keep yourself hydrated and keep the nausea at bay.
- Take deep breaths in fresh air, since it can calm your stomach.
- Eat snacks with a lot of carbohydrates between meals.
- Avoid having an empty stomach, since hunger pangs can cause nausea.

- Rest when tired and make sure to get enough sleep.
- Learn which types of food cause nausea and vomiting and which food will help alleviate morning sickness. Every woman is different and what doesn't work for others might work for you.
- If you feel sick, chew on fresh ginger or suck on a slice of lemon.
- Remember that if the nausea is severe and continues past the 14th week of your pregnancy, you might need medical assistance.

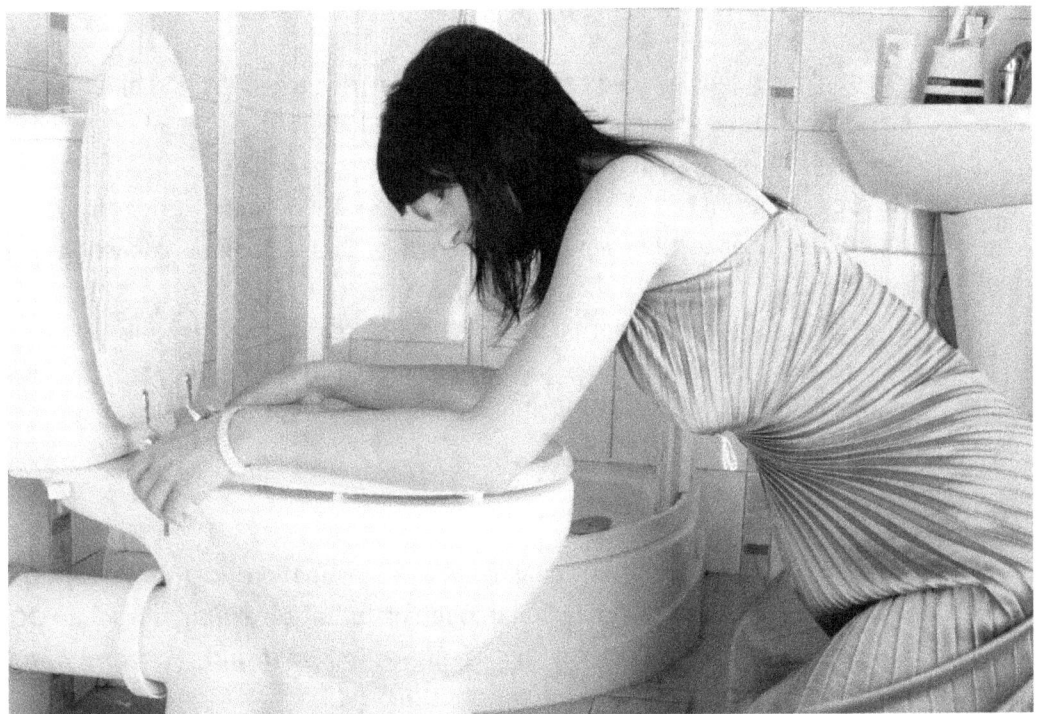

## HEARTBURN

Pregnant women often experience heartburn, which can be very uncomfortable and sometimes even painful. The reason heartburn is more common during pregnancy is that the hormonal changes in your body slow down your body's digestive system, and your growing uterus putting pressure on your stomach may contribute to this. Heartburn can be helped by the following:

- Eat small and frequent meals so as not to overload your digestive system.
- Avoid food that might upset your stomach such as spicy food, caffeine, chocolate and cola, as well as fried and fatty foods.
- Avoid wearing tight clothes, not just for comfort but for giving your stomach extra room to stretch.

- Try to lie down for a while after each meal.
- Sleep on a pillow or elevate your head by using blocks underneath the feet of the bed.

## CONSTIPATION

Constipation is common during pregnancy and is most often caused by the hormonal changes in your body. Sometimes it can also be caused by the iron supplements in your prenatal vitamins since a high level of iron in your body can lead to constipation. Reduce the risk of constipation by taking the following actions:

- Hot drinks can help a lazy digestive system, so drink a healthy herbal tea or a glass of warm water containing lemon juice with your breakfast.
- Drink plenty of water, at least 10 glasses of fluids every day.
- Eat food with a lot of fiber to kick start your digestive system, such as fruits, vegetables, fiber-fortified cereals, whole-wheat bread, legumes and whole-grain products.
- Olive oil, yogurt and dried fruit can help against constipation as well.
- If you suffer from severe constipation, you should consult your doctor about the appropriate remedy (be careful about taking any drugs to treat constipation, such as Senna).

Another method I find useful in dealing with constipation is using the Image Visualization technique. I use the image of an opening lotus flower with the sound OOO. You can read more about it in my book: ***Childbirth without Fear: A Simple Technique to Conquer Your Childbirth Fears Quickly.***

## EDEMA

Edema is the accumulation of fluids between the cells in your body, outside the blood vessels. It results in swelling, especially in the legs. Take the following actions to alleviate the swelling:

- Limit your salt intake since salt can worsen the edema. Stay away from spicy or salty food, as well as processed food and junk food which contain large amounts of sodium.
- Drink a lot of water. It may sound counterintuitive, but having a lot of water in your body increases your circulation and helps your body transport the liquid away from your legs.

- Increase your potassium intake. The mineral potassium can reduce the accumulation of edema fluid and increase the secretion of excess fluid from the body. A combination of excessive sodium and potassium deficiency is found in many people who suffer from hypertension. Among the best sources of potassium are apples, asparagus, cabbage, oranges, tomatoes, bananas, seaweed kelp and alfalfa.

*When Andrea became pregnant with her second child, she had a severe case of morning sickness. Every morning she would throw up the little breakfast she had, and as soon as she had eaten lunch her body returned all of the nutrients. It was the same with dinner, and Andrea was losing weight quickly.*

*Then a friend of hers told her that grains, vegetables and ginger could help against the nausea. It was also recommended that Andrea eat small meals several times daily instead of three big ones. After only a few days of eating according to these new tips, Andrea was feeling a lot better. She was able to keep down her meals and lost a lot less nutrients through vomiting. In the end she was able to regain her energy and have a healthy pregnancy without further issues.*

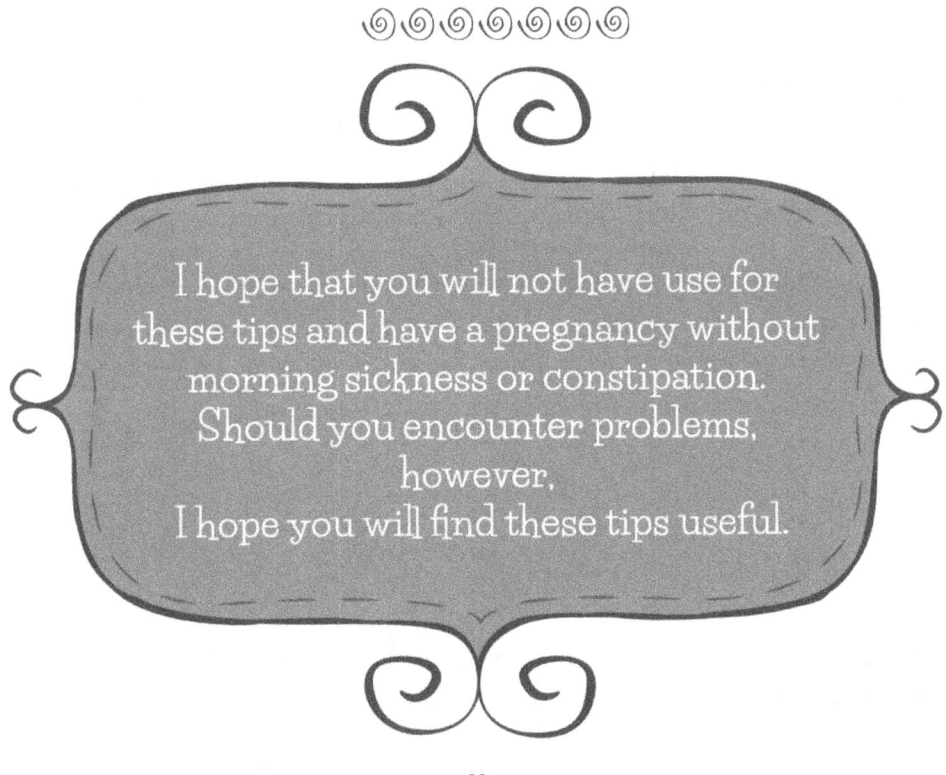

I hope that you will not have use for these tips and have a pregnancy without morning sickness or constipation. Should you encounter problems, however, I hope you will find these tips useful.

# CHAPTER 11- SUMMARY

I want to thank you for taking the time to read and learn about how to prepare healthy food during your pregnancy. Now I hope that both you and your baby can enjoy the benefits of a healthy diet.

The book took you through the steps of finding the easiest and simplest ways to eat healthy food. The first step of eating healthy is changing your own attitude towards healthy food, and you were given some tools that should help you along the way. If you lack motivation or find eating healthy a challenge, you can use several methods to get you back on track.

You have learned the importance of nutrition during your pregnancy and what ingredients your baby needs to ensure his healthy development. Some kinds of food should be avoided while you're pregnant, since they could contain bacteria or substances which may be harmful to your baby. Other kinds of food are recommended, and you were given some tips on how to get the nutrients your baby needs.

Finally, you learned some tips for preparing a healthy diet all week without taking up too much of your time. Preparing healthy food doesn't have to be difficult or time consuming if you cook according to the Concentrated Effort method. You also found out how food can help you with common problems that may arise during pregnancy.

Now you can go through your pregnancy with a healthy diet which provides both you and your baby with the nutrients you need. When it is time to give birth, you will have given your child the best possible chances for a healthy life. Your new diet may even help you during labor by giving you more energy and strength.

All that is left for you to do is start cooking and eating healthy meals. Prepare your menus in advance, cook as often as suits your schedule and eat tasty and nutritious food.

Remember that every day you do not eat healthy food, you may be robbing your growing baby of vital nutrients he needs for healthy growth.

I wish you a wonderful pregnancy filled with energy and well-being brought on by a healthy diet. I also wish you a happy and easy birth.

*"Always do your best. What you plant now, you will harvest later."*

*- Og Mandino (author)*

I would love to hear what you thought about this book. Please stop by  and review it at:

# Bonus Chapter - How to strengthen your mind

Eating healthy during pregnancy depends a lot on your state of mind and your own attitude. The attitude is affected by your mind.

Our mind is our most powerful tool when it comes to dealing with stress, anxiety and fear. Using only our mind, we can turn a negative outlook into a positive one and rid ourselves of worries. The problem is, most often we don't know how to use our minds to the fullest extent. Only when we learn to do so, can we enjoy the benefits of a strong, confident mind.

Our minds are constantly influenced by what we see, hear and read every day. Some people let every impression enter straight into their minds, and some know how to sort between what is good and what is bad for them. The difference between these people is their awareness of how things influence them.

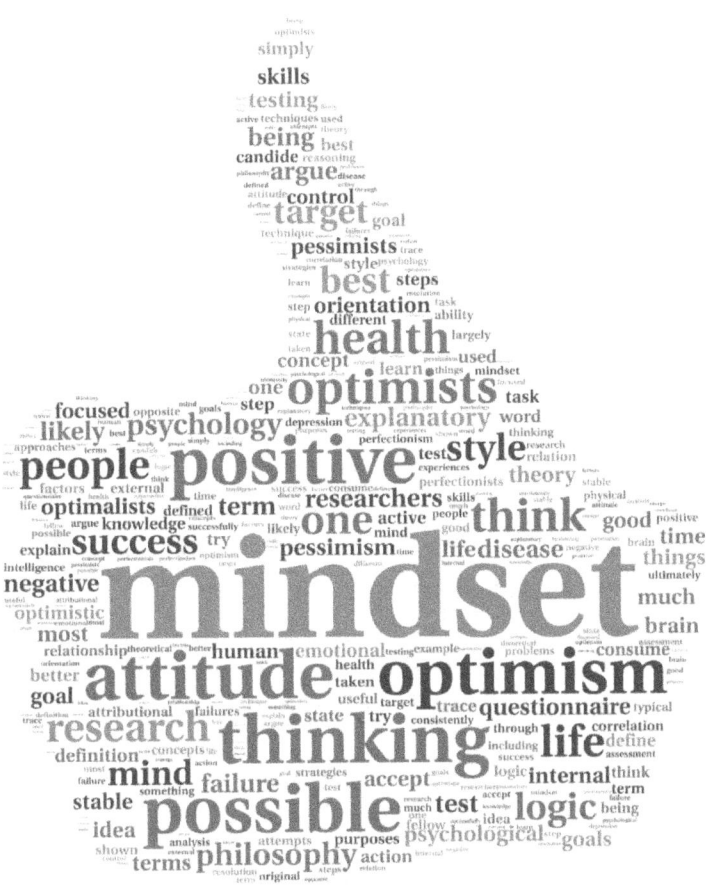

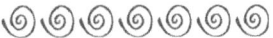

*Mariah came into contact with people who told of frightening tales of pregnancy and childbirth, every day, while she was working at a hospital. Women told her what had gone wrong and how painful labor was. When Mariah became pregnant with her first child, she found those stories difficult to ignore. The result was a stressful pregnancy because she worried every day that something would go wrong.*

*During labor, Mariah was terrified about the pain and became very tense. The result was that her contractions were much more painful than necessary. Only after a while did she realize that the pain wasn't as bad throughout her pregnancy as she had thought it would be. She began to relax and found that she didn't need to worry about it as much. In the end, she had a fast and uncomplicated delivery of a healthy baby boy.*

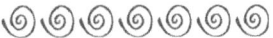

Worry brings unnecessary stress and tension. You can rid yourself of all of this by learning more about the powerful tools that will help you strengthen your mind. Minimize bad influences and expose your mind to positive images. The more you can control your mind, the easier it will be to get what you want.

After a healthy pregnancy and a natural birth of my first child, I realized that I owed much of my success to the way I managed my mind. I decided to learn more about the mind, which is a very powerful tool, and use my newly-acquired technique on other aspects of my life.

During my quest of learning more about the mind, I encountered a great mentor, Bob Proctor. Bob is a talented speaker who teaches professional coaching seminars and his work focuses on helping people harness the power of their mind to succeed in their lives. He is also a teaching master of the Law of Attraction, which stipulates that focusing on positive thoughts can bring a positive outcome.

I had participated in a number of his seminars which were the start of a big change in my life. The most important lesson for me was **that repetition is important when talking about the mind.**

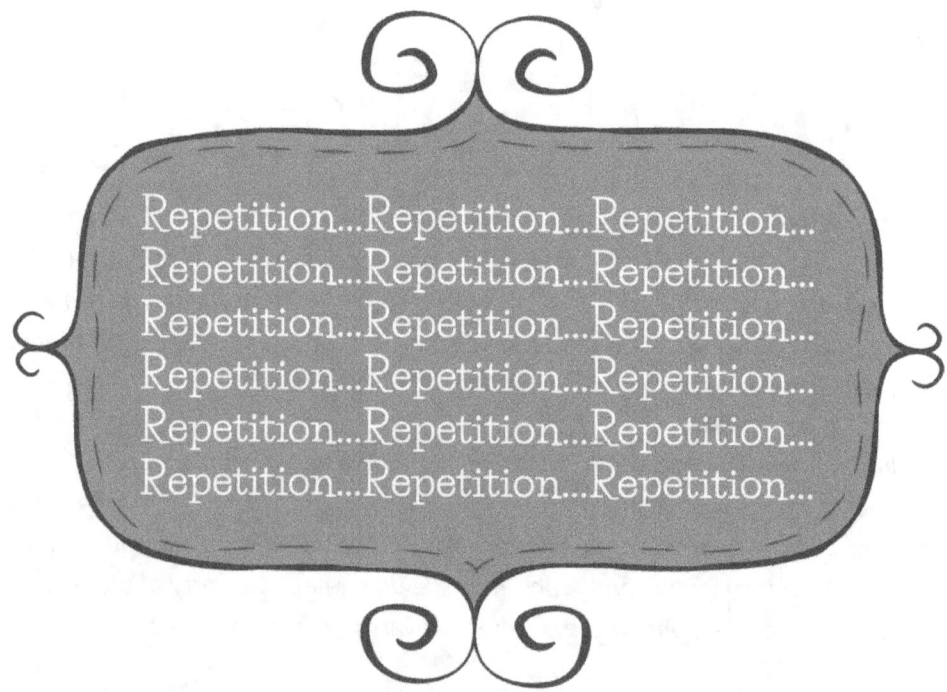

Repetition can be done in several ways:

1. Listen to audio lessons while driving in your car or doing exercises, etc. I made it a habit to listen to one lesson, every day. Usually I listened to each lesson 30 days in a row in order for it to sink into my mind and become a part of it.

An audio which I can greatly recommend is "The Strangest Secret" by Earl Nightingale. This is one of the most influential messages on audio, and it explores the question of what it takes to succeed in the ever-changing world of today.

2. Get a positive insight every day. This is a powerful tool to grow your own awareness and learn more about your mind. I like to open my day with "Insight of the Day" by Bob Proctor. By signing up for a daily insight, you will receive a short message that will give you something positive to focus on.

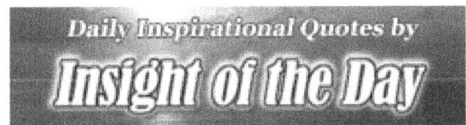

3. Participate in weekly sessions of learning new information about the mind. I signed up for Bob's streaming club. In this club I have the opportunity to meet him once a week, to learn the most efficient and valuable lessons about the mind. I've found that attending the weekly meetings is like going to a "mind gym."

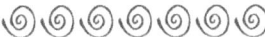

*My friend Sophia had a difficult first pregnancy and suffered from a wide variety of symptoms as well as post-partum depression. When she became pregnant with her second child, she was determined to change her mindset and have a positive experience during pregnancy and childbirth. She signed up for Bob Proctor's daily insight, attended his weekly seminars and listened to every audio book on the subject that she could find, while driving to work every day. When it was time for her childbirth she felt relaxed and at ease. The delivery went very well, without complications, and this time around, she didn't suffer from depression.*

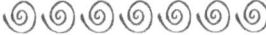

I hope you will find these tools helpful and that you now know where to begin in your quest to expand your mind and to find more positive influences. This will help you throughout the challenging time that is pregnancy and childbirth. Afterwards, you and your baby will be able to reap the benefits of your training, since you will have a more positive outlook and a strong mind, free from negative thoughts and unnecessary worries.

*"You are today where your thoughts have brought you; you will be tomorrow where your thoughts take you."*

*~James Allen (author)*

**You can find two more helpful tools in my other books:**

*Childbirth without Fear: A Simple Technique to Conquer Your Childbirth Fears Quickly*

*How to Reduce Pregnancy Stress Using the Positive Affirmations Technique*

# ABOUT THE AUTHOR

Einat is a mother to a lovely girl.
She has been studying for the last 15 years the powerful ways to use your mind &
subconscious and live a quiet, peaceful and better life.
She tries to live according to the methods she's learned in all areas of her life.

Einat believes in the principles of flow , liberation and positive thinking.
That's why she loves the shape of the spiral.
She implements these principles in her daily life.
She's on an endless journey of her personal development and tries to do the best she
can.

When she became pregnant with her first daughter, she implemented the tools she
learned about herself in order to have an easy, pleasant and empowering pregnancy.
Einat had many concerns about the birth process but with the tools and techniques
which she applied to herself she was able to overcome these concerns and gave a
natural childbirth to a healthy daughter.

Einat is the co-founder of a new pregnancy web site www.myPregnancyToolkit.com that
brings a set of practical tools for pregnant women that focuses on the pregnancy issues
from the mind's perspective.

### Your success means a lot to me.

If you have a comment or question, please contact me at my email address:

contact@myPregnancyToolkit.com

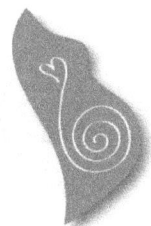 **My Pregnancy Toolkit**
Simple Tools for Busy Women that will Enable You
to Enjoy an Easy Pregnancy and Childbirth

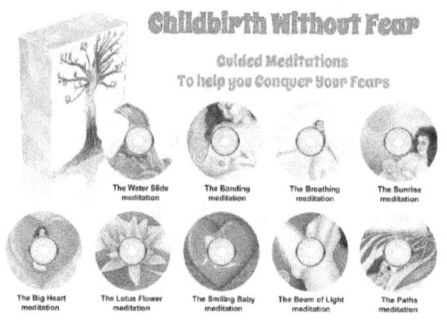

## Childbirth without Fear - Guided Meditations to help you Conquer Your Fears

The *audio guided meditations* are part of a set of helpful tools that can help you eliminate your upcoming childbirth fears. These meditations can serve as a stand alone tool and also as a complement to the book *Childbirth without Fear: A Simple Technique to Conquer Your Childbirth Fears Quickly*. They are easy to practice and can be used any time and anywhere.

The audio guided meditations are available on Amazon.

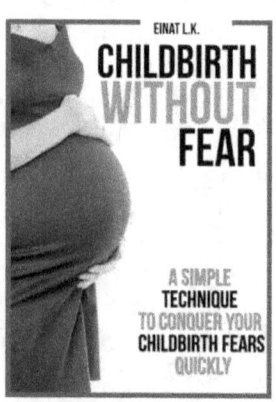

## Childbirth without Fear: A Simple Technique to Conquer Your Childbirth Fears Quickly

In this book you will learn about the image visualization technique and how it can help you eliminate your upcoming childbirth fears. It will help you reduce your stress and you'll even begin to enjoy your pregnancy. This technique can effectively replace your fearful mental images of childbirth with those that are reinforcing and positive.

The book is available on Amazon.

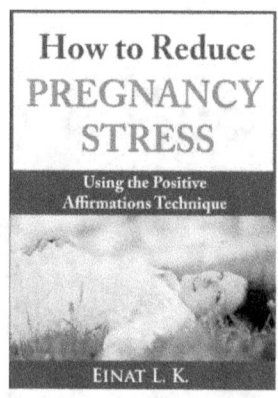

## How to Reduce Pregnancy Stress Using the Positive Affirmations Technique

In this book you will learn about the positive affirmations technique and how it can give you and your baby a happy, healthy glow inside and out and reduce the stress you might feel during your pregnancy.

The book is available on Amazon.

www.ingramcontent.com/pod-product-compliance
Lightning Source LLC
Chambersburg PA
CBHW081239280526
45787CB00006B/2717

* 9 7 8 1 6 3 0 2 2 0 6 8 6 *